CSCS Study Guide 2023-2024

Complete Review + 660 Test Questions and Detailed Answers Explanations for the NSCA Certified Strength and Conditioning Specialist Exam (3 Full-length Exams)

Copyright 2023 by Newstone Test Prep - All rights reserved.

Printed in the United States of America

Newstone Test Prep is not affiliated with any official testing organization. All test names and registered trademarks belong to the owners or related official testing organizations.

This book is geared towards providing precise and reliable information about the topic. This publication is sold with the idea that the publisher is not required to render any accounting, officially or otherwise, or any other qualified services. If further advice is necessary, contacting a legal and/or financial professional is recommended.

From a Declaration of Principles that was accepted and approved equally by a Committee of the American Bar Association and a Committee of Publishers' Associations.

In no way is it legal to reproduce, duplicate, or transmit any part of this document, either by electronic means, or in printed format. Recording this publication is strictly prohibited, and any storage of this document is not allowed unless with written permission from the publisher. All rights reserved.

The information provided herein is stated to be truthful and consistent, in that any liability, in terms of inattention or otherwise, by any usage or abuse of any policies, processes, or directions contained within, is the solitary and utter responsibility of the recipient reader. Under no circumstances will any legal responsibility or blame be held against the publisher for any reparation, damages, or monetary loss due to the information herein, either directly or indirectly.

Respective authors own all copyrights not held by the publisher.

The information herein is offered for informational purposes solely, and is universally presented as such. The information herein is also presented without contract or any type of guarantee assurance.

The trademarks presented are done so without any consent, and this publication of the trademarks is without permission or backing by the trademark owners. All trademarks and brands within this book are thus for clarifying purposes only and are owned by the owners themselves, and are not affiliated otherwise with this document.

CSCS® and Certified Strength and Conditioning Specialist® are registered trademarks of the National Strength and Conditioning Association, which neither sponsors nor endorses this product. Newstone Test Prep is not affiliated with the National Strength and Conditioning Association.

Table of Contents

Introduction 6
    Functions of a Certified Strength and Conditioning Specialist 6
    Education Requirements 7
    Career Options 9
    Remuneration 10
    Traits of a Successful CSCS 11
    Difference Between a Strength and Conditioning Coach and a Personal Trainer 11
    Pros and Cons of Becoming a Certified Strength and Conditioning Specialist 12

Chapter 1: The CSCS Exam 13
    Eligibility Requirements 13
    How to Register for the Exam 13
    What to Expect on Exam Day 14

Chapter 2: Basic Scientific Foundations: Exercise Science; Overview of Muscle Anatomy and Physiology 20
    Neuromuscular Anatomy and Physiology 31
    Anatomy and Physiology of the Neuromuscular System 32
    Bone and Connective Tissue 34
    Basic Principles of Biomechanics 38
    Bioenergetics and Metabolism 44
    Bioenergetics 48
    Neuroendocrine Physiology 54
    Cardiopulmonary Anatomy and Physiology 56
    Physiological Adaptations to Exercise, Training, and the Impact of Recovery Strategies 71
    Special Consideration of Differences Among Athletes 78
    Scientific Research and Statistics in the Exercise Sciences 80

Sports Psychology 81
Psychological Foundations of Performance 83
Motor Learning and Skill Acquisition Techniques 86
Indicators of Mental Health Issues in Athletes 89
Causes of Mental Health Issues in Athletes 90
Nutrition 90
Effects of Hydration Status and Electrolyte Balance/Imbalance on Health and Performance 102
Effects, Risks, and Alternatives of Common Supplements 104
Performance-Enhancing Substances and Methods 107
Impact of Alcohol and Drugs on Performance 111
Effects of Performance Enhancing Drugs on Performance 112

Chapter 3: Practical and applications 114
Exercise Technique 114
Program Design 147
Organization and Administration 168
Testing, ongoing monitoring, and data evaluation 182

Test 1 Questions 189
Test 1 Answers and Explanations 265
Test 2 Questions 324
Test 2 Answers and Explanations 400
Test 3 Questions 466
Test 3 Answers and Explanations 543

Introduction

Certified Strength and Conditioning Specialists (CSCS) are professionals who train athletes by using scientific knowledge with the end objective of enhancing their athletic performance.

Functions of a Certified Strength and Conditioning Specialist

<u>Training</u>

Certified strength and conditioning specialists design and implement training sessions for athletes to enhance their speed and agility, strength, power, flexibility, and balance. They also ensure these training sessions are safe and effective.

<u>Designing Conditioning Programs</u>

A strength and conditioning specialist designs and implements a comprehensive conditioning program using research-driven scientific principles to improve the overall flexibility and endurance of athletes. They are also responsible for determining the intensity and duration of the exercise best suited for an individual. Most conditioning specialists also offer nutritional advice as a part of their conditioning program.

<u>Maintenance of Weight Machines and Conditioning Equipment</u>

In addition to designing and implementing conditioning programs and training, strength and conditioning specialists are responsible for ensuring used equipment is functional and that the conditioning facility is in good shape. They also establish policies and procedures in accordance with the NSCA Strength and Conditioning Professional Standard Guideline to ensure the smooth and safe operation of the facility.

Rehabilitation

Strength and conditioning specialists collaborate with a physical therapist to design a program to prepare a rehabilitating athlete to get back to base-level health. The focus is on building up the strength, endurance, and flexibility of an athlete following injury.

Conducting a Needs Analysis

Strength and conditioning specialists also work together with the athlete's sports coach to conduct an in-depth analysis of their performance to assess how effective a training program is, as well as determine the strengths and weaknesses of each individual athlete.

Education Requirements

Obtain a Bachelor's Degree

Most strengthening and conditioning roles require a minimum of a bachelor's degree. To begin your career in this field, you will need to obtain a bachelor's degree in exercise, kinesiology, or another exercise-related field like physical education.

Consider a Graduate Degree

While a graduate degree is not mandatory, it is becoming increasingly common as many job listings have a master's degree in an exercise science or related field as a preferred qualification for applicants. If you are looking to stand out from a pool of applicants, consider getting an advanced degree in exercise physiology, sports nutrition, exercise and sport science, or even physical therapy (doctorate).

Obtain CPR/AED Certification

The National Strength and Conditioning Association (NSCA) requires that a strength and conditioning specialist obtain CPR and automated external defibrillator (AED) certification before they can be certified as a strength and conditioning specialist.

The American Heart Association and the American Red Cross both offer the recommended CPR/AED certification courses. To enroll, you may reach out to these organizations and find an upcoming course in your area. Keep in mind that for these courses to be accepted, they must include a practical hands-on session.

Take Accredited Certification Exams

Credentials are critical to becoming certified as a strength and conditioning specialist. Many job postings ask that applicants have at least one certification. You can get certified by completing credentialing programs such as the NSCA Certified Strength and Conditioning Specialist Certificate or the Strength and Conditioning Coach Certified Certification (SCCC) from the Collegiate Strength and Conditioning Coaches Association.

Volunteer at a Collegiate or Professional Sports Program

It is important to get practical hands-on experience to help you stand out in your application. Consider volunteering with an expert, a local sports team, or a community center to gain experience within the field, even prior to employment.

Attend Conferences and Symposiums

It is not enough to have a bachelor's degree and stop there; in order to stay relevant in this field, you must stay up to date on current evidence-based techniques and routines in exercise sciences. Attending conferences, workshops, or symposiums is one way to learn the most relevant and latest techniques from experts, which can help bridge the gap between theory and practice. Such events also provide you with an opportunity to network with other professionals.

Career Options

Strength and Conditioning Coach

A strength and conditioning coach is one of the most common paths for people with a certification in strength and conditioning. As a strength and conditioning coach, you're responsible for training athletes and assisting them in improving their strength, endurance, balance, and speed. You provide personalized training and decide what practice is best for each athlete. You are also responsible for ensuring that the techniques used are safe so that the athletes do not sustain injuries. Strength and condition coaches may also provide nutritional advice to athletes.

Athletic Director

You can explore an administrative position with your certification in strength and conditioning. One way to do this is to become an athletic director at a college or university. As an athletic director, you will be responsible for managing the athletic program operations, including budget allocation, hiring, pre-season game planning, dispute resolution, and ensuring overall department efficiency.

Exercise Physiologist

With a certification in strength and conditioning, you can work as an exercise physiologist in hospitals, fitness centers, or rehabilitation clinics. In this role, you will be responsible for using evidence-based methods to improve athletes' overall health and performance. You are in charge of designing and administering stress tests, creating personalized workout plans, and developing safety programs that reduce the likelihood of injuries while participating in sports.

Physical Therapists

You can also pursue a career as a sports physical therapist; however, this is a less-common path. As a physical therapist, you will be in charge of developing programs that prevent sports-related injuries. You could also work in a rehab clinic, developing exercise plans to help injured athletes recover faster and with less pain. You will monitor the athlete's progress and make necessary adjustments to the plan. You could assist athletes with injuries ranging from sprained ankles to strokes in resuming their daily activities.

Assistant Professor

As a certified strength and conditioning specialist, you can also consider a career in academia. As an assistant professor in strength and conditioning, you will be responsible for teaching exercise science or kinesiology courses to college or university students. You will also be in charge of grading student work, training teaching assistants, and developing course material for your class.

Remuneration

As of November 2022, the average salary for a strength and conditioning specialist is $46,845. However, your salary may vary depending on your education, certification, and years of experience. The typical range is between $40,006 to $54,113. Salary may also differ depending on location and expertise.

San Francisco has some of the highest-paid certified strength and conditioning specialists, with a median salary of $74,617, 51% higher than the national average. Other states with highly paid strength and conditioning specialists include Minnesota, Massachusetts, New York, Rhode Island, New Jersey, and Vermont.

Traits of a Successful CSCS

- Ability to evaluate and correctly analyze information

- Outstanding leadership abilities

- Ability to form strong interpersonal relationships

- Close attention to details

- Ability to communicate effectively and clearly, both verbally and in writing

- Strong moral principles (integrity and honesty)

- Ability to take the initiative

Difference Between a Strength and Conditioning Coach and a Personal Trainer

<u>Education</u>

A high school diploma or GED is typically required for a career as a personal trainer, although some personal trainers pursue an associate's or bachelor's degree in order to gain a competitive advantage.

A bachelor's degree in exercise science, kinesiology, or physical education is the minimum requirement for a strength and conditioning specialist. The majority of strength and conditioning specialists also have a graduate degree.

<u>Certification</u>

Personal trainers and strength and conditioning coaches must obtain certification in their field after completing the educational requirements.

The National Strength and Conditioning Association offers certifications to strength and conditioning coaches. You can also obtain certification from the National Academy of Sports Medicine's performance enhancement specialist certification, the International Sports Sciences Association's ISSA strength and conditioning coach certification, and the Collegiate Strength and Conditioning Coaches Association's strength and conditioning coach certification.

Personal trainers can become certified through a variety of organizations, including the American Council on Exercise (ACE) Personal Trainer Certification, the American College of Sports Medicine (ACSM) Personal Trainer Certification, and the National Council on Strength and Fitness (NCSF) Personal Trainer Certification.

Pros and Cons of Becoming a Certified Strength and Conditioning Specialist

Pros

- Flexible schedule.
- Increased job satisfaction.
- Network and meet new people.
- Work with athletes of all backgrounds.

Cons

- Difficult clients.
- Unsteady income.
- Increased risk of injury.
- Long work hours.

Chapter 1: The CSCS Exam

Eligibility Requirements

Before registering for the CSCS examination, you should have the following:

- Academic transcripts: bachelor's degree or higher
- CPR/AED certification

How to Register for the Exam

Registration

To register for the exam, visit the NSCA website and create an account. Once your account is created, you will receive your customer ID number. You will then be required to log in, confirm your eligibility, and complete the registration form. You must submit all required documents (including eligibility verification) as well as a $25 application fee.

Approval

Once your application is approved, you will proceed to schedule your preferred date for the exam. At this time, you must pay your exam fees, which are $340 for NSCA Student and Professional Members and $475 for non-members.

Scheduling an exam

You will receive an email within 2-3 business days after completing your registration. This email will include instructions for scheduling your exam appointment. You can schedule your exam either online or over the phone by calling a customer service representative.

Rescheduling an exam

If you are unable to make it to your exam appointment, you can reschedule free of charge within the authorization period. However, you can only schedule exams on the available testing dates.

Application fees

The CSCS exam has a $25 application fee. After that, you must pay the exam fee. The exam fee is $340 for NSCA Student and Professional Members, and $475 for non-members.

Retake policy

If you are dissatisfied with your results, you may retake the exam 90 days after your most recent attempt. However, if you have a job offer that depends on you getting an NSCA certification, or if your scaled score on your last attempt was 63% or higher, you might be able to request a waiver of the 90-day waiting period. Keep in mind, this waiver is only available once.

What to Expect on Exam Day

Preparation

1. Have your form of identification ready (passports, driver's licenses, or any government-approved ID). Photocopies or ID cards that have already expired will not be accepted.

2. Arrive at the testing center at least 15–30 minutes prior to your appointment.

Mode of exam delivery

The CSCS exams are conducted as multiple-choice, computer-based tests at designated centers.

Exam length

The CSCS exam has 220 questions, not all of which are scored. Only 190 questions will be counted toward your final score. The time limit for the scientific foundation question is 90 minutes, while the time limit for the applied/practical section is 2 hours and 30 minutes. This exam has a total time limit of four hours.

Exam breaks

The CSCS exam allows for a 15-minute break between exam sections, which does not count against exam time. If you take breaks outside of this time, the exam timer will continue to run. During these scheduled or unscheduled breaks, you are not permitted to access any personal items or devices.

Exam format

The CSCS exam has 220 multiple-choice questions divided into two sections: the Scientific Foundation section and the Practical/Applied section. Only 190 out of 220 questions are scored.

The first section will test students in nutrition, biomechanics, and sports psychology. The second section will test students on techniques, evaluation, and program management.

It is important to note that the unscored questions do not contribute to your total score; rather, they are used by the exam administrator to determine future exam questions. You will not know which questions are scored.

Exam complexity

The CSCS exam is regarded as moderately difficult, with a pass rate of 57% on average. The questions are written at various levels of complexity. The CSCS exam tests the following: recall, application, and analysis.

Recall questions test your knowledge of concepts, principles, facts, and methods.

Application questions require situation-specific knowledge. These types of questions include basic calculation and your ability to identify the relationship between concepts.

Analysis questions require you to examine multiple variables to determine the best response. These questions require complex calculations and identification. Many test takers may consider analysis questions the most difficult because they require the combination of several concepts to solve a problem.

How exams are scored

After your exam, you will receive two scores—raw and scaled. Your raw score is determined by the number of correctly answered questions. Your performance, however, is measured by your scaled score. To pass the certification exam, you must obtain a scaled score of 70 or higher.

What to do if Your Scores are Canceled

If an individual is deemed ineligible, the NSCA Certification Committee may cancel exam scores. Candidates who are found to be ineligible will not have their registration fees refunded. You may, however, file a written appeal with the certification committee. The basis for the appeal, as well as any relevant documents, should be included in your appeal. You must also pay a $25 appeal fee. If your appeal is successful, this fee will be refunded.

Test Accommodations

To ensure that all candidates have equal opportunities, the NSCA committee makes special accommodations for people with documented disabilities. This accommodation is only valid for one examination. You must request accommodations for each exam.

To request accommodation, fill out the accommodation request form and provide supporting documentation.

Rules and Regulations

1. Do not bring personal items (including cell phones, PDAs, calculators, and watches) into the examination room. You will receive your writing supplies at the testing center.

2. If you are more than 15 minutes late to your exam, you may be permitted to take the test only at the testing center's discretion. Note that the registration fee will be forfeited if you do not show up on time or do not withdraw or cancel your registration.

3. You must obtain permission from the exam supervisor before leaving the examination room.

4. You are not permitted to ask questions concerning the exam's content. However, you are allowed to ask your questions using the comment function built into the exam software.

Test Results

Your score results are made available immediately after the exam. The official score report will be available for download on your Pearson VUE account 24 hours after the completion of your exam.

Tips on How to Pass the CSCS Exams

Start studying early: The secret to success in any exam is to begin studying as soon as possible.

Set a target date: When planning your study time, set dates for when you should have mastered specific concepts and for reviewing what you have learned.

Get good study material: One of the best ways to do well on the CSCS exam is to have good study material that covers all of the NSCA's topics.

Review the question bank: Before you begin studying in depth, go over the question banks in your study guide to see how well you understand certain concepts.

Exam prep class offered by NSCA: Attend in-person clinics offered by experienced professionals familiar with the exam to get a thorough review of the exam content.

Get some practical experience: Hands-on experience would be beneficial in the practical/applied section. This is because the CSCS exam assesses your capacity to apply your knowledge, skills, and abilities to practice as a strength and conditioning professional.

Commit to a study schedule: Choose a time when you can study with utmost concentration and stick to it. You do not need to study for long periods of time; instead, stick to the study schedule you have established.

Practice: After reading through the study guide and reviewing the content, it is critical to practice the study guide questions. You can start with an untimed session to assess your performance, then set your timer to complete each set of 220 questions in four hours.

How to choose the right resource material

The NSCA does not recommend any CSCS exam study materials. However, some of the best materials are those that adhere to a detailed content outline of the exam topics and include enough practice questions with detailed explanations of answers. Review the content outline of each study guide and ask colleagues which materials helped them the most to choose the best material for you.

How to improve your recall

The best way to remember information is to first understand the content of the material you are reading rather than simply memorize or cram the concept. Once you've grasped the material, try to relate the information you need to remember to something you're already familiar with. You can also try making flashcards and mnemonics to help you become more familiar with the information and improve recall. Research shows that reviewing material before going to bed helps to solidify the information learned.

How to be organized

1. Set the exam date on a calendar and then work backwards to plan your study.

2. Schedule your study time using a physical or online planner.

3. Always keep your study table or area clear of clutter.

4. Maintain your study schedule.

5. Set specific objectives for each study session.

6. Schedule breaks and time to run other programs.

Chapter 2: Basic Scientific Foundations: Exercise Science; Overview of Muscle Anatomy and Physiology

Introduction to the Muscular System

There are over 600 muscles in the human body. These muscles are responsible for movement, digestion, respiration, and even sight. There are three types of muscle: skeletal muscle, cardiac muscle, and smooth muscle.

<u>Functions of Muscles</u>

- Create force and enable movement

- Control voluntary movement

- Contribute to the stability and maintain posture

- Regulate respiration

- Enable digestion

- Enable proper oxygenation

- Control heartbeat

- Regulate temperature

- Control urination

<u>Characteristics of Muscles</u>

- Excitability: Muscles are excitable. This means they have the ability to react to stimuli.

- Contractility: Muscles can contract or shorten.

- Extensibility: Muscles can stretch or extend.

- Elasticity: Muscles can return or rebound to their original length when relaxed.

Types of muscle tissue

Skeletal muscle: In humans, skeletal muscles make up about 30 to 40 percent of the total body weight. Skeletal muscles are voluntary and control movements. The skeletal muscle is attached to the bones through the tendons.

Skeletal muscles appear striated under the microscope. The striated appearance is due to the arrangement of the microfilaments, which are crossed with repeating patterns of red and white lines.

Skeletal muscles are multinucleated and comprise individual fibers bundled together to form muscle spindles. A single muscle fiber is mostly made up of actin and myosin fibers that are surrounded by a cell membrane (sarcolemma).

There are two major classes of skeletal muscles: Type I, also known as slow oxidative, and type II also known as fast-twitch.

Cardiac muscle: The cardiac muscle, also called myocardium, is an involuntary muscle only found in the heart. This muscle is also striated and surrounds the heart chambers.

Cardiomyocytes are the muscle cells found in the heart. Each cardiomyocyte is made up of cytoskeletal and contractile elements that are linked together by intercalated discs.

The cardiac muscle, like the skeletal muscle, has contractile units known as sarcomeres. However, unlike skeletal muscles, cardiac muscle fibers have only one nucleus and shorter fibers.

The cardiac muscles are responsible for the contraction of the heart, and thus, pumping blood into various blood vessels. The cardiac muscles contain specialized cells called pacemaker cells. Pacemakers generate the electrical impulses that cause the heart to beat.

Smooth muscle: The smooth muscle is an involuntary muscle responsible for digestion, micturition (urination), and even the regulation of blood flow. This muscle cell is found in the walls of the lungs, reproductive organs, skin, blood vessels, eyes, and the GIT.

Unlike skeletal and cardiac muscle, the smooth muscle is not striated; rather, its cells are arranged in sheets, giving it a smooth appearance.

The cytoplasm of smooth muscle contains a large number of actin and myosin fibers, which are responsible for contraction. The sarcoplasmic reticulum is another important structure found in smooth muscle that helps to sustain contraction.

Microscopic Anatomy of Skeletal Muscle

Skeletal muscles appear striated under the microscope. These muscle cells have long, multinucleated fibers that are unbranched and wide. The multinucleated fibers are composed of myofibrils. Myofibrils are protein fibers made up of actin and myosin filaments, responsible for contraction.

Sarcomeres are the functional units of muscle cells and are responsible for contraction. Muscle contracts when sarcomeres found within many myofibrils crosslink and pull on each other, causing the sarcomere to shorten. The sarcomere has three bands: the A band and two I bands. The dark region of a striation contains thick myosin filaments and is referred to as the A band, while the lighter region contains thinner actin filaments and is referred to as the I band.

Fascicles are bundles of skeletal muscle fibers. The fascicles are surrounded by the perimysium. The endomysium, on the other hand, surrounds a single muscle fiber, while the epimysium surrounds the collection of fascicles that comprise a single muscle.

The plasma membrane of a muscle fiber is called the sarcolemma, which contains the sarcoplasmic reticulum.

Gross Anatomy of the Skeletal Muscle

1. Muscles of the head and neck

Muscles found in the face include the frontalis, buccinator, orbicularis oris, laris oculi, and zygomaticus. These muscles control a wide range of facial expressions.

The temporalis muscle, medial pterygoid, lateral pterygoid, and masseter are responsible for chewing or mastication. These muscles are connected to the mandible and are among the strongest in the human body.

Some of the muscles found in the neck include the sternocleidomastoid, the suprahyoid muscles, platysma, scalene muscles, and the infrahyoid muscles. These muscles allow the head to move in all directions.

2. Muscles of the trunk

The muscles of the trunk control important body functions such as breathing, defecation, micturition, and movement.

The muscles of the trunk can be broadly categorized as follows:

3. The anterior trunk muscles:

• Muscles of the thoracic cage: Muscles in the thoracic include the pectoralis major, pectoralis minor, the intercostal muscles, subcostal, serratus anterior, and transversus thoracis muscles.

- Muscles of the abdominal wall: Muscles found in the abdominal part of the anterior trunk include pyramidalis, external abdominal oblique, internal abdominal oblique, transversus abdominis, and rectus abdominis. These muscles are involved in flexion and rotation of the trunk.

The rectus abdominis is the muscle found at the front of the pelvis between the ribs and the pubic bone. This muscle is commonly referred to as a "six-pack" in athletic individuals.

The transversus abdominis is the deepest flat muscle. When the transverse abdominis contracts, it compresses the abdominal organs and assists expiration.

4. Posterior trunk muscles (muscles of the back):

- Superficial muscles of the back: The muscles found in these regions include the trapezius, latissimus dorsi, rhomboid major and minor, serratus posterior superior and inferior muscles, and levator scapulae.

- Deep muscles of the back: These include the erector spinae muscles, multifidus muscle, semispinalis capitis, longissimus, spinalis, splenius capitis muscle, and iliocostalis.

5. Muscles of the upper extremity

Muscles in the upper extremity include the trapezius, brachioradialis, coracobrachialis muscle, biceps brachii, triceps brachii, flexor carpi radialis muscle, deltoid, subclavius muscle, supraspinatus muscle, and pronator teres muscle.

6. Muscles of the lower extremity

The muscles of the lower extremities include the tibialis anterior muscle, vastus medialis, vastus lateralis muscle, biceps femoris muscle, quadratus femoris muscle, adductor brevis muscle, obturator internus muscle, fibularis brevis, quadriceps, gluteus maximus, gluteus minimus, gluteus medius, iliopsoas, hamstring, and the adductor muscles of the hip.

The quadriceps femoris muscle, located in the thigh, is responsible for straightening the leg at the knee, while the hamstring muscles flex the knee.

The gluteal muscles, also referred to as the glutes, comprises three muscles: gluteus maximus, gluteus minimus, and gluteus medius. The gluteal muscles adduct the thigh. The iliopsoas muscle flexes the thigh. It is important for walking and running.

Physiology of the Muscular System

The muscular system is responsible for movement. The muscle is derived from the mesoderm and is made up of specialized cells called muscle fibers. It is muscle fibers that are responsible for contraction. Within the muscle fibers are myofibrils. Myofibrils are rod-like organelles containing sarcomeres. Sarcomeres are the basic functional unit of the muscle cells. Sarcomeres consist of thick myosin filaments and thin actin filaments.

Muscle contraction begins when the action potential reaches the end of the axon of a motor neuron at the neuromuscular junction. When the action potential reaches the end of the axon, acetylcholine, a neurotransmitter is released, which triggers a chain reaction that activates voltage-gated calcium ions, thus causing calcium influx into the sarcoplasm. This calcium influx causes the myosin heads to crosslink with the actin so that muscle contraction can begin. As this happens, ATP is hydrolyzed.

This contraction causes the sarcomeres in surrounding myofibrils to crosslink, delivering a power stroke, which causes the myofibrils to become shorter, thus, pulling the entire muscle and causing it to become shorter. As long as there is enough calcium in the sarcoplasm to bind to troponin, and ATP is available, the muscle will continue to contract. A muscle will stop contracting when the calcium is pumped back into the sarcoplasmic reticulum, or when ATP stores are depleted and the muscle cells are fatigued.

Types of Muscle Contraction

- Isometric contraction: "Iso" means the same, and "metric" means length. An isometric contraction is a type of muscle contraction in which the length of the muscle remains unchanged. In this type of contraction, the muscle does not shorten during contraction. Isometric contraction is the type of muscle contraction that occurs when an individual needs to grip an object, not when moving a heavy object prior to lifting.

- Isotonic contraction: "Iso" means the same, and "tonic" means force/tension. Here, the force (tension) remains the same while the muscle length changes. This type of contraction requires more work and force than isometric.

There are two types of isotonic contraction:

1. Concentric contraction: In this contraction, the muscle fibers shorten while the muscle contracts. This type of contraction occurs when an individual bends their arm at the elbow or when they lift weight toward the shoulders.

2. Eccentric contraction: Here, the muscle fibers lengthen or elongate as they contract. An example of this type of contraction occurs when an individual lowers a weight slowly under tension.

Isotonic vs. isometric exercise

Isotonic exercise, sometimes called aerobic or endurance exercise, involves high-repetition movements against low resistance. Examples of isotonic exercise include walking, swimming, running, and cycling.

Isometric exercise, also called resistance or strength training, involves low-repetition movements against high resistance. Examples of isometric exercise include weightlifting or strength training.

Types of Muscle Fibers

Based on physiological functions, there are three different types of muscle fibers:

1. Slow oxidative fibers: Also called slow-twitch or type I fibers. They relatively contract slowly and use aerobic respiration (oxygen and glucose) to produce ATP.

Slow-twitch fibers are usually small and have a rich supply of mitochondria and blood capillaries. They usually appear red in fresh tissue because of their high myoglobin content.

The slow-twitch fibers are resistant to fatigue, making them ideal for prolonged postural activities such as standing. The deep back muscles responsible for posture are primarily composed of Type I slow oxidative fibers.

Endurance athletes (marathons, cross-country runners, long-distance cyclers, triathlons, and endurance swimmers) tend to have more slow-twitch fibers.

Type I muscle fibers have low force production.

2. Fast oxidative glycolytic fibers: Also called type IIa fibers. They are relatively fast and also use aerobic respiration to generate ATP.

These fibers also contain many mitochondria like the type I fibers. However, they also have large amounts of glycogen, which makes them capable of anaerobic respiration.

The type IIa fibers do not possess significant myoglobin; hence, they appear lighter in color than type I fibers.

The type IIa fibers are more fatigue resistant than the type IIx fibers and are thus used in movements that require sustained energy. These fibers belong to the fast-twitch-fatigue resistant units. Type IIa fibers produce intermediate force.

Competitive swimmers usually have high amounts of type II fibers. In addition, athletes who specialize in strength and power sports, such as sprinters and weightlifters, possess a higher proportion of type IIa fibers in their muscles.

3. Fast glycolytic fibers: Also called IIx fibers, type IIb, or fast-twitch fibers. They have fast contractions and primarily use anaerobic glycolysis to produce ATP.

These fibers usually appear white because they have a poor supply of blood capillaries. These fibers are large and poor in mitochondria.

Fast glycolytic fibers are utilized to generate swift and forceful muscle contractions for quick and powerful movements.

Type IIx fibers are more prone to fatigue than type I and type IIa fibers. These fibers belong to the fast-twitch-fatigue prone units. Splinters have an abundance of type IIx fibers. Type IIx fibers produce high force.

All or none's law

According to this principle, if a motor unit is stimulated with an intensity that is sufficient to produce a response, all of the muscle fibers innervated by that motor unit will contract simultaneously and with maximal force.

Musculoskeletal System

Skeletal system

The skeletal system is broadly divided into two: the axial skeleton and the appendicular skeleton.

The axial skeleton comprises the cranium (skull), vertebral column (ranging from vertebra C1 to the coccyx), ribs, and sternum.

The appendicular skeleton is made up of the pectoral girdle (shoulder girdle), the pelvic girdle (formed by the left and right innominate bones or coxal bones), and the bones in the limbs.

Joints

A joint is the location where two bones connect with each other. Joints can be categorized either by the type of connective tissue that dominates histologically or by the degree of movement allowed functionally.

Histologically, there are three types of joints in the human body. They include fibrous, cartilaginous, and synovial joints.

- Fibrous joint: In fibrous joints, bones are connected by fibrous tissue, which is primarily composed of collagen. These joints are typically rigid and immovable (classified as synarthroses) and lack a joint cavity. This includes joints in sutures of the skull.

- Cartilaginous joints: Here, the bones are connected by either hyaline or fibrocartilage. These joints are further divided into two categories based on the type of cartilage present: primary cartilaginous joints and secondary cartilaginous joints. Primary cartilaginous joints are composed solely of hyaline cartilage. They may be slightly flexible or immovable. Secondary cartilaginous joints contain either hyaline or fibrocartilage and are slightly moveable. This includes intervertebral disks.

- Synovial joints: These joints are the most significant joints in terms of function, as they are highly movable (diarthroses) and allow for a wide range of motion. Examples include the elbow and knee.

Levers

In the human body, a lever is a system that applies force at one end (the fulcrum) to lift an object at the other end (the load). The bones, muscles, and joints in the human body form a system of levers that work together to produce movement.

These levers work by utilizing a rigid structure (bone) as a support, with a force acting upon it (muscle) to create a rotational movement (angular motion) around a fixed point (joint), the fulcrum. The load or resistance being lifted or moved is placed on the rigid structure and can include the weight of the body part being moved and any additional weight it may be carrying.

There are three classes of levers:

1. First-class lever: In this type of lever, the fulcrum is located between the effort (muscle force) and the load. An example of this type of lever can be seen in tricep extension.

2. Second-class lever: Here, the load is located between the effort and the fulcrum. This type of lever is found in the ankle. An example is a standing heel raise.

3. Third-class lever: In this type of lever, the effort is in the middle between the fulcrum and the load. This type of lever is seen during a biceps curl.

To easily recall the order of the levers, you can use the acronym "FLE" to remember which part of the lever is positioned in the center.

For a first-class lever, the fulcrum is in the middle.

In a second-class lever, the load is situated in the middle.

For a third-class lever, the effort is in the middle.

Neuromuscular Anatomy and Physiology

Introduction to the Neuromuscular System

The neuromuscular system is a combination of the nervous system and the muscular system.

The nervous system is made up of the central nervous system and peripheral nervous system. The central nervous system is made up of the brain and spinal cord.

The peripheral nervous system is divided into the somatic system and the autonomic system. The somatic nervous system stimulates muscle activation, while the autonomic nervous system can either stimulate or inhibit muscle activation. The autonomic nervous system is further divided into the sympathetic and parasympathetic nervous system.

The muscular system, on the other hand, is made up of skeletal muscle, cardiac muscle, and smooth muscle.

How Does the Neuromuscular System Work?

Neurons are the basic functional unit of the nervous system. Neurons relay messages from the brain to various parts of the body by means of electric signals. There are three kinds of neurons: sensory, motor, and interneurons. Motor neurons are responsible for sending electrical signals from the brain to the muscles.

Motor neurons are located close to muscle fiber. The junction between a motor neuron and muscle fiber is called the neuromuscular junction. When the motor neurons release a chemical known as acetylcholine, the muscle fiber picks up a signal, which tells the muscle fiber to contract.

<u>The Neuromuscular Junction</u>

The neuromuscular junction (NMJ) is the junction between the motor neuron and motor fiber. It is where the motor nerve ending makes a synapse with muscle fibers, causing the fibers to contract and movement to occur.

The neuromuscular junction is made up of three types of cells: The nerve terminals, glial cells—also called the perisynaptic Schwann cells—and muscle fibers.

Inside the nerve terminals are synaptic vesicles that contain acetylcholine. The acetylcholine is usually released when the electrical impulse at the nerve terminals triggers calcium influx.

The perisynaptic Schwann cells participate in the development, maintenance, and repair of the synapse.

Anatomy and Physiology of the Neuromuscular System

Motor axons: These are nerve fibers that carry signals from the spinal cord to effector organs. Axons are usually longer than dendrites.

Dendrites: Dendrites are nerve fibers that receive signals from other cells. Dendrites are usually short and branched.

Motor fibers: These are nerve fibers that carry signals that stimulate muscle contraction. They are also referred to as efferent fibers.

Motor neurons: This is a neuron that carries motor impulses from the central nervous system to effectors. Motor neurons have single axons and multiple dendrites.

Muscle spindles: Muscle spindles are also called stretch detectors, as they detect changes in the length of a muscle. They are able to sense the rate of change in muscle length.

Synaptic end bulb: This is the rounded area on the end of the axon terminals. It contains the synaptic vesicles in which acetylcholine is stored. When the synaptic end bulb receives electrical signals, it stimulates the influx of calcium.

Synaptic cleft: This is a small space between the presynaptic neuron and the postsynaptic cell. It is often referred to as the final component of the NMJ.

Acetylcholine: This is the chief neurotransmitter in the parasympathetic nervous system. It helps neurons communicate with other cells.

Acetylcholinesterase: This is the enzyme responsible for breaking down acetylcholine. It breaks down acetylcholine into acetic acid and choline. This enzyme is found at the postsynaptic neuromuscular junctions in muscles.

Adaptation of the Neuromuscular System to Exercise

Some factors that affect how the neuromuscular system adapts to exercise include the type of exercise, the frequency of exercise, the intensity of exercise, and the duration of exercise.

The skeletal muscle adapts to mechanical overload by increasing the size of the muscle. It does this by forming new proteins and increasing the number and size of muscle fibers.

Strength training will increase muscle size and strength by improving myofibrillar protein synthesis. On the other hand, endurance training usually targets aerobic metabolism and thus will improve fatigue resistance.

Bone and Connective Tissue

The human skeleton contains 206 bones, not including teeth and sesamoid bones. The bones in the human body are broadly divided into two: axial bones and appendicular bones.

There are 80 axial bones. Axial bones are found in the head, ribs, sternum, ears, and trunk.

There are 126 appendicular bones. This includes the bones in the arms, shoulders, hands, legs, ankles, feet, and hips.

<u>Classification of Bones</u>

Bones can be classified into four major types:

Long bones: These types of bones are longer in one direction and have a long shaft with two knob-like structures at both ends or extremes. These bones are longer than they are wide. They consist primarily of compact bones, with spongy bones at their extremes. Long bones are found in the arms, thighs, legs, and forearms.

Short bones: These types of bones are shaped roughly as a cube, with their length and width approximately equal. They consist primarily of spongy bones, although the outer surface is covered in a thin layer of compact bone. Short bones are found in the wrist and ankle.

Flat bones: Flat bones are usually thin, flattened, and slightly curved. They are made up of a layer of spongy bone placed in between two compact bones. The bones in the skull and ribs are flat bones.

Irregular bones: These types of bones vary in shape and do not fit completely into any of the above classifications. Irregular bones may have flat, notched, or ridged surfaces. The bones in the vertebrae and skull are irregular bones.

Bone Cells

There are three main types of bone cells in the human body:

• Osteoblasts: These bone cells are involved in bone formation and mineralization.

• Osteoclasts: Osteoclasts function opposite that of osteoblasts. Osteoclasts are responsible for breaking down bone and bone tissue resorption.

• Osteocytes: Osteocytes are sometimes referred to as "inactive" osteoblasts. These bone cells are responsible for regulating bone formation and breakdown.

Bone remodeling

Bone remodeling is the process of replacing an old bone with a new bone. This process regulates bone replacement after an injury such as a fracture.

Osteocytes and osteoclasts both contribute to bone remodeling. The osteoclasts will resorb old bone tissues at various sites, whereas the osteoblasts aid in the formation of new bones in order to maintain skeletal structure.

Connective Tissues

Connective tissues are a group of tissues that provide support and maintain form in the body. As their name implies, these tissues also connect different organs in the body. Connective tissues can be found in every part of the body—between muscle cells, tissues, and organs. Connective tissue arises from the mesoderm. These tissues are made up of protein fibers, cells, and ground substances.

Types of Connective Tissues

Connective tissues can be differentiated based on the types of cells present or the structure. Some important connective tissues include:

Loose connective tissue: The loose connective tissue, also called areolar tissue, is the body's most abundant type of connective tissue. These tissues can be found in the outer part of the esophagus, blood vessels, nerves, and organs.

Loose connective tissues are made of an extracellular matrix and also collagen, elastin, and reticular fibers. However, the fibers in this connective tissue are not tightly packed together.

These tissues attach epithelial tissues to adjacent tissues. They are the main site of fluid and gas exchange between the blood and surrounding tissues. They also protect internal organs like blood vessels and nerves.

Dense fibrous connective tissue: Dense connective tissue protects the internal organs and holds the bones and muscles. Unlike loose connective tissues, the dense collagen fibers are tightly packed.

Dense connective tissue can be regular or irregular. The fibers in dense, regular connective tissues follow a consistent pattern and are arranged parallel to one another. The primary function of these tissues is to provide mechanical support to muscles and other organs. Examples of dense regular tissues include tendons and ligaments. On the other hand, the dense irregular tissues have a woven appearance and are mainly made up of collagen fibers. These tissues surround and protect internal organs, bones, and some types of cartilage from injury. They also provide support for the skin. Dense irregular connective tissues can be found in the dermis (the skin), spleen, and liver. These tissues can also be seen in the brain (dura mater).

Adipose tissue: Adipose tissues are fat-filled tissues. They help store energy and conserve body heat. They also help maintain insulin sensitivity and regulate glucose. Depending on where it is found, there are two types of adipose tissue: subcutaneous fat and visceral fat. The subcutaneous fat is found under the skin, while the visceral fat is found in-between internal organs like the kidney and eyeballs.

Adipose tissue is also classified into white and brown adipose tissue based on its function. Under the microscope, the white adipose tissue appears as a large unilocular lipid droplet. It helps store excess energy and insulates the body from extreme temperatures. Under the microscope, the brown adipose tissue is seen as multiple small lipid droplets. It generates heat by consuming energy reserves in the body. This type of tissue is often found in infants and decreases with age. It helps protect infants from hypothermia.

Elastic connective tissue: These connective tissues contain elastic fibers called elastin. Elastin is responsible for the elastic nature of these tissues. Structures made up of elastic connective tissues can return to their original position after stretching. These can be found in tissues in the lungs and the walls of large arteries. They can also be found in the skin layer, ligaments, and tendons.

Cartilage: The cartilage is a strong and flexible connective tissue. These types of connective tissues can be found almost anywhere two bones meet in the body. For example, these tissues can be found in the growth zones of the bones, in the external ear, and between the ribs and sternum. The cartilage helps to cushion and facilitate joint movement, absorb shocks, and lubricate joints. They also help keep the airways open.

There are three types of cartilage in the body: hyaline cartilage, elastic cartilage, and fibrous cartilage.

Osseous tissue (bone): The osseous tissue, also called bone tissue, is a mineralized connective tissue that provides physical support and structure to the body. The osseous tissue is made up of both organic and inorganic components. The main inorganic component is calcium phosphate, in the form of a mineral called hydroxyapatite. These compounds help make the body's skeleton stronger. The main organic components of the osseous tissues are the collagen fibers, which offer elasticity in these tissues.

Blood: Blood is a connective tissue that contains a fluid matrix known as plasma. Unlike other connective tissues, blood tissue has no fibers. It is mainly made of water and solutes. Blood helps in the transportation of oxygen and the regulation of body temperature.

Blood comprises erythrocytes (red blood cells), leukocytes (white blood cells), and platelets. The process through which these cells are produced in the bone marrow is called hematopoiesis.

Basic Principles of Biomechanics

Biomechanics is the study of the structure, movement, and function of biological systems. There are five basic components of biomechanics. These are motion, force, levers, momentum, and balance.

<u>Principles of Biomechanics</u>

There are eight basic principles of biomechanics.

1. The principle of force-motion

This is the first principle in biomechanics, and it is based on Newton's first law of motion. It states that before motion can occur, some forces must act first. According to this principle, an unbalanced force acts on our bodies when we initiate or modify movement.

2. The principle of force–time

This principle is also known as the impulse-momentum principle. Newton's second law of motion underpins the force-time principle.

According to this principle, the greater the time force is applied, the greater the resulting motion.

Mathematically, this law is written as: impulse = force (mass x acceleration) x time

3. The principle of inertia

Inertia is the tendency of objects or bodies to resist any attempt to change their motion. The principle of inertia measures how difficult it is to change an object's state of motion. According to this principle, the heavier the object, the more force is required to change its motion.

4. The principle of range of motion

The range of motion principle refers to the type of motion used to create movement. The range can be specified by linear or angular motion of the body segments.

Angular motion is the movement of body parts or objects around an axis, while linear motion is the movement of a body/object in a straight line.

According to this principle, increasing the range of motion increases the speed of a motion. We can also limit the range of motion to gradually slow down a motion that started fast.

5. The principle of balance

Balance is related to stability. It is the ability to control the body position in relation to the base of support of an object.

Two key terms to note in balance are:

• Centre of gravity: This is an imaginary point where the total body mass is concentrated.

• Centre of mass: This is the body's balancing point. It is the actual point where the body mass of the body is concentrated.

6. The principle of coordination continuum

According to this principle, the goal of the movement determines the optimal timing of muscle actions or segmental motion.

When the movement's goal involves high forces, more simultaneous muscle actions and joint rotations are required; for instance, high-intensity basketball free throws or weight lifting. Whereas for high-speed/low-force movements, more sequential muscle and joint actions are required.

7. The principle of segmental interaction

This principal states that energy in a system of linked bodies can be transferred across body segments and joints.

8. The principle of optimal projection

There is an optimal range of projection angles for most human movements involving projectiles. In simpler terms, this principle refers to the angle, velocity, and height of release an object needs to be projected to achieve a specific goal.

Mechanical Advantage

This measures the efficiency of a system and is calculated by dividing the length of the moment arm for the applied force by the length of the moment arm for the resistive force.

When the mechanical advantage is greater than one, it means that the applied force (muscle force) is smaller than the resistive force, but still generates the same amount of torque.

On the other hand, when the mechanical advantage is less than one, it is considered a disadvantage, as the applied force must be greater than the resistive force to generate the same amount of torque.

The patella and mechanical advantage

The patella (knee cap) enhances the performance of the quadriceps muscle group by keeping the tendon away from the center of rotation at the knee. Without the patella, the tendon moves closer to the center of rotation, causing the muscle's mechanical advantage to decrease. This is because the length of the moment arm, which represents the distance from the joint axis of rotation to the line of action of the tendon, affects the muscle's mechanical advantage.

Moment arm and mechanical advantage

The moment arm changes as the lifted weight changes its horizontal distance from the elbow during arm flexion. Most muscles in the body work at a disadvantage, leading to higher forces within the muscles and tendons during physical activities compared to the force exerted on external objects or the ground.

Anatomical Planes of the Human Body

A body is said to be in an anatomical position when it is in an upright position, with the arms hanging down by the sides and facing forward.

- The sagittal plane divides the body into left and right sections.

- The frontal plane separates the body into front and back parts.

- The transverse plane cuts the body into upper and lower sections.

Biomechanical Factors in Human Strength

The factors affecting human strength include:

- Neural control

- Muscle cross-sectional area

- Arrangement of muscle fibers

- Muscle length

- Joint angle

- Muscle contraction velocity

- Joint angular velocity

- Strength-to-mass ratio

- Body size

Neural control: This refers to the number of motor units involved in a contraction, the size of these units, and the rate of firing.

Muscle cross-sectional area: The force exerted by a muscle is related to its cross-sectional area, not its volume.

Arrangement of muscle fibers: The arrangement of muscle fibers can vary, with pennate muscles having obliquely aligned fibers and non-pennate muscles having fibers aligned along the tendon.

Muscle length: Muscle strength is greatest when the muscle is at its resting length. The amount of torque generated depends on muscle length, leverage, type of exercise, joint, muscles used, and speed of contraction.

Strength-to-mass ratio: The strength-to-mass ratio is important in sports such as sprinting and jumping, and for determining an athlete's relative strength compared to others in their weight class.

Body size: Body size has an impact on strength, with larger bodies having a higher body mass relative to muscle strength.

Joint Biomechanics in Resistance Training

In general, the risk of injury from resistance training is low compared to other sports and physical activities.

Lower back

The lower back is prone to injury in resistance training. Hence, exercises should be performed with a slightly arched lower back.

The Valsalva maneuver and weightlifting belts increase intra-abdominal pressure and aid in supporting the vertebral column. A belt is not necessary for exercises not affecting the lower back but may be worn for near-maximal and maximal sets.

For people who do not want to wear belts, building strength in the back muscles and muscles generating intra-abdominal pressure is a reasonable alternative.

Shoulders

Shoulders are prone to injury due to their structure and the forces they are subjected to. To protect the shoulders, warm up with light weights, perform balance exercises, and control speed.

Knees

The knees are prone to injury due to their location between two long levers. To protect the knees, minimize the use of wraps.

Elbows and wrists

Overhead lifts pose the greatest risk to the elbows and wrists. However, the risk is low compared to other sources of injury in overhead sports.

Avoid epiphyseal growth plate damage by reducing stress on the posterior aspect of the elbow or distal radius.

<u>How to reduce the risk of injury</u>

- Warm up with light weights and perform a full range of motion of basic exercises.

- Avoid maximal loads without proper preparation and technique instruction.

- Incorporate variation and be mindful of pain.

- Take care when adding plyometric drills to the training program.

Bioenergetics and Metabolism

Bioenergetics is the study of energy flow in a biological system. It describes how macronutrients like carbohydrates, protein, or fat are converted into micronutrients like glucose or ATP.

<u>Metabolism</u>

Metabolism refers to the total sum of all chemical reactions in a biological system.

<u>Types of Metabolic Reactions</u>

Metabolic reactions can be broadly divided into two:

1. Catabolism: Catabolism is the breakdown of large molecules into small molecules. Catabolic reactions are usually exergonic reactions. This means they release energy into a system. This type of reaction breaks down energy-storing molecules such as lipids to release energy and make ATP.

Examples of catabolic reactions include respiration and digestion of food.

2. Anabolism: Anabolism is the buildup of large molecules from smaller ones. Anabolic reactions are often endergonic reactions, which require energy from the system. This type of reaction demands energy provided by ATP, NADH (nicotinamide adenine dinucleotide), and NADP.

Examples of anabolic reactions/pathways include the synthesis of large proteins from amino acid building blocks and the synthesis of DNA from nucleic acid building blocks.

Classes of Metabolic Reactions

There are three major classes of metabolic reactions:

- The Phosphagen System

Also called the ATP-CP system, it is one of the fastest ways to resynthesize ATP. This energy system is instantaneously available.

This system does not use carbohydrates or fat to generate ATP. Instead, creatine phosphate (CP) found in the skeletal muscles donates a phosphate to ATP to generate ATP.

The phosphagen system is anaerobic or oxygen-independent, as it does not require oxygen to resynthesize ATP.

This system of producing energy is convenient during short-term, intense activities that require a large amount of energy to be produced by the muscles. However, because there is a limited store of CP and ATP in the skeletal muscle, fatigue occurs easily.

This is also the main energy system used for all-out exercise, which lasts for about one to thirty seconds. It is the energy used for short-term, high-intensity exercise like sprinting or lifting weights.

- Glycolysis

This system is the second fastest way to resynthesize ATP. It involves the breakdown of blood glucose or muscle glycogen (carbohydrates) through a series of chemical reactions to form pyruvate.

When a molecule of glucose is broken down into pyruvate using glycolysis, two molecules of ATP are produced in the process.

Glycolysis produces little energy, however. Its only advantage is that energy is produced fast.

The pyruvate formed undergoes two main reactions after formation. It is either converted to lactate or to acetyl-CoA. If it is converted to acetyl CoA, the coenzyme will enter the mitochondria for oxidation and produce more ATP.

Glycolysis is the main system used for all-out exercises that last anywhere between 10 seconds to two minutes. Glycolysis is used during high-intensity, anaerobic exercises such as sprinting or weightlifting, which involve short, explosive bursts of activity. However, this system has limited capacity and produces lactate as a byproduct, causing fatigue and muscle soreness.

- The aerobic system

The aerobic system is dependent on oxygen, and it is the most complex of the three energy systems. It is also the slowest way to resynthesize ATP. However, it is responsible for most of the cellular energy produced by the body.

The aerobic system follows two major pathways: The Krebs cycle (also called the citric acid cycle or TCA cycle) and the electron transport chain.

The aerobic system uses blood glucose, glycogen, or fat to resynthesize ATP in the mitochondria of the muscle.

When using carbohydrates as a source of fuel, glucose and glycogen are first metabolized by glycolysis into pyruvate. The pyruvate formed is then used to synthesize acetyl CoA, which enters the Krebs cycle. From the Krebs cycle, electrons produced are transported to the electron transport chain, where ATP and water are formed.

For every glucose completely metabolized through glycolysis, Krebs cycle and electron transport chain, 36 molecules of glucose of ATP are produced.

Note that one glucose molecule produces a total of 38 ATP through the process of aerobic respiration, which is made up of ATP generated from glycolysis, the link reaction, the TCA cycle, and oxidative phosphorylation in the electron transport system.

Oxidative phosphorylation is the primary energy system at work when the body is at rest.

Using fat as an energy source

When using fat molecules as an energy source, triglycerides are first broken down into free fatty acids and glycerol.

The free fatty acid is then transported to the muscle mitochondria, where they form acetyl CoA. Just like with carbohydrates metabolism, acetyl is transported to the Krebs cycle.

In this process, electrons are moved to the electron transport chain to form ATP and water. This process, however, produces more molecules of ATP than the oxidation of glucose or glycogen.

Summary

- Activities lasting zero-to-six seconds are usually extremely high intensity, and the phosphagen system primarily supplies the energy.

- Activities lasting six-to-thirty seconds are usually very high intensity and the phosphagen and fast glycolysis system primarily supply the energy.

- Activities lasting thirty seconds to two minutes are usually high intensity and mainly supplied by fast glycolysis.

- Activities lasting two-to-three minutes are usually of moderate intensity and fueled mainly by fast glycolysis and the oxidative system.

- Activities that take longer than three minutes are usually low intensity, and energy is mainly provided by the oxidative system.

Bioenergetics

Bioenergetics is the study of energy changes that occur in living cells or how energy is transformed in living cells, tissues, and organisms.

Principles of Bioenergetics

There are two main principles of bioenergetics:

1. The first law of thermodynamics: The first law of thermodynamics is also referred to as the law of conservation of energy. It states that energy can neither be created nor destroyed, but it can be changed from one form to the other. This means that the total energy of any system is always constant.

Mathematically, this can be written as:

$\Delta U = Q - W$

Where,

ΔU = Change in the Energy

Q = Heat Added

W = Work done by the system

2. The second law of thermodynamics: The second law of thermodynamics states that energy flows from a higher energy level to a lower energy level—or heat moves from a hotter system to a colder one. According to this law, the entropy will always increase and cannot be negative.

Fundamental Concepts of Thermodynamics

The first and second laws of thermodynamics can be combined to give:

$\Delta H = \Delta G + T\Delta S$

This can be rearranged as

$\Delta G = \Delta H - T\Delta S$

Where,

ΔG = Gibbs Free Energy

ΔH = Change in enthalpy

ΔS = Change in entropy

T = temperature in kelvin

Here are some important concepts that you should know in thermodynamics:

Enthalpy: Enthalpy (H) is a measure of the total amount of thermal energy contained in a thermodynamic system. It is defined as the sum of the internal energy of a system (U) and the product of its pressure (P) and volume (V).

Mathematically, enthalpy is given as:

$H = U + PV$.

Entropy: Entropy (S) is a measure of the amount of thermal energy in a thermodynamic system that is unavailable for doing useful work. It is also defined as a measure of the disorder or randomness of a system.

Gibbs free energy (ΔG): Gibbs free energy is a quantity used to calculate the maximum amount of work done in a thermodynamic system when the temperature and pressure are constant. It is the amount of energy used by a system to get work done.

Gibbs free energy will tell us how spontaneous a reaction is. It can be defined mathematically as: $\Delta G = \Delta H - T\Delta S$.

If ΔG is negative, then the process is spontaneous, and the reaction is an exergonic reaction.

If ΔG is positive, then the process is nonspontaneous, and the reaction is endergonic.

And if ΔG is zero, then the process or the reaction is at equilibrium.

Thermodynamic systems: In thermodynamics, a system refers to the matter and its surroundings involved in energy transfers.

There are two types of systems: an open and a closed system. In an open system, both energy and matter can be transferred between the system and its surroundings.

On the other hand, a closed system is one that does not allow the transfer of matter to its surroundings. However, in this system, energy can flow in and out of the system.

Thermodynamic states: Thermodynamic state is a set of values used to identify the condition of a system at any given time. The state of a system can be identified by the volume, temperature, and pressure.

Thermodynamic equilibrium: This is a state in which the properties of a system do not change with time or spontaneously. In thermodynamics, a system is said to be in equilibrium when there is physical, thermal, mechanical, and chemical equilibrium.

Thermodynamic work: This is the quantity of energy transferred from one system to another, or from a system to its surroundings.

Exothermic reactions: This is a type of chemical reaction where energy is released as heat into the environment.

Endothermic reactions: This is a type of chemical reaction where energy is absorbed from the environment.

Some formulas you should know:

Power = Work / Time

Work = Force x Distance

Sample Calculation

If it takes an athlete 20 seconds to lift a 100 kg barbell two meters for six repetitions, what is the power output?

To calculate the power output, we need to use the formula:

Power = Work / Time

Where Work is the amount of energy expended in lifting the weight, and Time is the duration of the lifting activity.

To find the Work, we can use the formula:

Work = Force x Distance

where Force is the force required to lift the weight, and Distance is the distance over which the weight is lifted.

Since the weight is lifted vertically against gravity, we can find the force using:

Force = Weight x Gravity

Where Weight is the mass of the weight being lifted, and Gravity is the acceleration due to gravity.

We know that:

Weight = 100 kg Gravity = 9.81 m/s^2 Distance = 2 m Repetitions = 6 Times = 20 seconds

So, the force required to lift the weight is:

Force = Weight x Gravity = 100 kg x 9.81 m/s^2 = 981 N

And the work done in each repetition is:

Work = Force x Distance = 981 N x 2 m = 1,962 J

Therefore, the total work done in 6 repetitions is:

Total Work = Work x Repetitions = 1,962 J x 6 = 11,772 J

Now, we can calculate the power output:

Power = Total Work / Time = 11,772 J / 20 s = 588.6 watts

Therefore, the power output of the athlete is 588.6 watts.

Bioenergetic Limiting Factors in Exercise Performance

The ranking of bioenergetic limiting factors in exercise performance is dependent on the intensity of the exercise.

Light marathon: Here, muscle glycogen is the most probable limiting factor, followed by liver glycogen and fat stores.

Moderate 1,500m run: Muscle glycogen and liver glycogen are the main limiting factors, while fat stores play a minor role.

Heavy 400m run: Liver glycogen is the most probable limiting factor, while muscle glycogen and fat stores play a similar role.

Very intense activity (e.g., discus throwing): Muscle glycogen and liver glycogen are equally limiting, while fat stores and ATP/creatine phosphate play a minor role.

Very intense repeated activity: For a very intense repeated activity such as ten repetitions of the snatch exercise at 60% of 1RM, muscle glycogen and ATP/creatine phosphate are the main limiting factors, followed by liver glycogen and fat stores. The pH level is also likely to decrease with increasing exercise intensity.

Interval Training

Interval training is a workout technique that aims to enhance the efficiency of energy transfer within the metabolic pathways, allowing predetermined periods of exercise and rest.

Work-to-rest ratios: The ideal work-to-rest ratios of various energy system includes:

- Phosphagen: Work-to-Rest Ratios of 1:12 to 1:20

- Fast Glycolysis: Work-to-Rest Ratios of 1:3 to 1:5

- Fast Glycolysis and Oxidative: Work-to-Rest Ratios of 1:3 to 1:4

- Oxidative: Work-to-Rest Ratios of 1:1 to 1:3

Neuroendocrine Physiology

Neuroendocrinology is the branch of biology that studies the relationship between the nervous system and the endocrine system. The main site of neuroendocrine interaction is the hypothalamus and pituitary.

By using resistance training, the endocrine system can be naturally influenced to boost growth in specific bodily tissues, resulting in improved performance.

Synthesis, Storage, and Secretion of Hormones

Hormones are chemical messengers produced, stored, and released into the bloodstream by the endocrine glands and some other cells.

The hypothalamus, pituitary gland, thyroid gland, parathyroid glands, heart, liver, adrenal glands, pancreas, kidneys, testes in males, and ovaries in females are among the primary glands and organs that secrete hormones.

Muscle and Hormone Interactions

The hormonal system, as part of an interconnected signaling network, impacts the metabolic and cellular changes in muscle due to resistance training.

Hormones also play a significant role in the protein synthesis and breakdown processes involved in muscle adaptation to resistance exercise.

Categories of Hormones

There are three main categories of hormones: steroids, peptides, and amines.

Steroids: These hormones are fat soluble and can cross the cell membrane. Examples include testosterone, progesterone, and cortisol.

Peptides: These hormones are not fat-soluble and thus cannot cross the cell membrane. Examples are growth hormones and insulin.

Amines: They are synthesized from the amino acid tyrosine (e.g., epinephrine, norepinephrine, and dopamine) or tryptophan (e.g., serotonin).

Hormones, Muscle Tissue Growth, and Remodeling

The three primary hormones involved in muscle tissue growth and remodeling include:

- Testosterone

- Growth hormone (GH)

- Insulin-like growth factors (IGFs)

Testosterone

Testosterone is a primary androgen hormone that interacts with skeletal muscle tissue, leading to increased strength and size of muscles, improved protein synthesis, and higher muscle mass.

Men experience diurnal testosterone variations, with exercise being more effective in the later part of the day. Women have lower concentrations of testosterone with little variation.

Large muscle group exercises result in a short-term increase in testosterone levels in men. In addition, a higher total testosterone level results in a higher potential for free testosterone, which is the hormone that interacts with target tissues.

Women have much lower concentrations of testosterone than men (15-20 fold lower), and any increase in testosterone after a resistance workout is small.

Growth hormone (GH)

Growth hormone (GH) is a hormone produced by the pituitary gland that interacts with various target tissues such as bones, immune cells, muscles, fat cells, and the liver.

GH release is regulated by neuroendocrine feedback and secondary hormones and can be altered by factors like age, gender, sleep, nutrition, alcohol, and exercise.

The response of GH to exercise stressors, including resistance exercise, depends on factors such as load, rest, and volume.

Women usually have higher GH levels and concentrations compared to men; however, this varies with the menstrual phase.

Insulin-like growth factors (IGFs)

Exercise results in acute increases in blood levels of IGF-I.

The variations in IGF-I appear to be influenced by the baseline concentrations prior to physical activity. If the baseline levels are low, IGF-I will increase, but if the baseline levels are high, there will be no change or a decrease in IGF-I.

Cardiopulmonary Anatomy and Physiology

The cardiopulmonary system involves the heart and the lungs. The word "cardio" refers to the heart, and the word "pulmonary" refers to the lungs. Therefore, the cardiopulmonary system explores the interrelationship between the heart and the lungs.

The role of the cardiopulmonary system is to regulate the flow of blood between the lungs and the heart.

The main function of the lungs is respiration (gaseous exchange), while the main function of the heart is to pump blood to all parts of your body.

Anatomy and Physiology of the Respiratory System

The respiratory system is made up of the airways, alveolus, lungs, thorax, and diaphragm. The function of each of these organs will be briefly explained.

The airway is also referred to as the respiratory tract. It is the parent name of all organs that allow airflow during respiration.

The airways are broadly divided into two: The upper and the lower airways.

The Upper Airways or Upper Respiratory Tract

The upper airway is made up of the nose, oral cavity, larynx, and pharynx. These organs act as a conductor of air. They also help to prevent foreign materials from entering into the trachea. In addition, they are actively involved in speech and smell.

In addition to the nose being an organ of smell, the primary function of the nose is to filter air. The inspired air then passes through the nasal cavity into the pharynx.

The pharynx, also known as the throat, is a hollow tube that starts from the nose and ends at the beginning of the esophagus and trachea. The larynx has both respiratory and digestive functions.

The pharynx is divided into three parts: nasopharynx, oropharynx, and laryngopharynx.

The nasopharynx can be found between the posterior portion of the nasal cavity and the superior portion of the soft palate.

The oropharynx is located between the superior portion of the soft palate and the inferior base of the tongue.

The laryngopharynx lies between the base of the tongue and the opening of the esophagus.

The larynx, also called the voice box, is a hollow tube that allows air to pass from the pharynx into the trachea. It is also responsible for the generation of sounds for speech.

Another important function of the larynx is its protective function against the aspiration of liquids and solids. At the opening of the larynx is a special flap of cartilage called the epiglottis. The epiglottis only opens to allow the passage of air into the airway. It closes to prevent food from entering into the airway during swallowing, thus preventing aspiration.

The Lower Airway or Lower Respiratory Tract

The lower airways consist of the lungs, alveoli, trachea, bronchi, and bronchioles. They are also referred to as the tracheobronchial tree, due to the branching structure of the airways that supply air to the lungs.

Trachea: This is a long, U-shaped tube made of cartilage that connects the larynx to the lungs. It is also known as the windpipe. The trachea divides into two main bronchi—one for each lung. The main function of the trachea is to allow air to pass in and out of the lungs during respiration.

Bronchi: These are two large tubes that carry air from the trachea (windpipe into the lungs). There are two main bronchi, one in the left lung, and the other in the right lung. The bronchi branch into smaller passageways that resemble three branches until they finally end at the alveoli.

Bronchioles: These are the smallest branches in the bronchial airways. They branch off from the main bronchi and serve as airways inside the lungs. The bronchioles have a diameter of around 1 mm and do not have any supporting cartilage skeletal structure.

Lungs: These are the main organs of the respiratory system. There are two lungs in the human body, and they are further sectioned into lobes. The right lung has three lobes and the left lung has two lobes. The right lung is also slightly larger than the left lung.

The lungs are separated by a compartment called the mediastinum and covered by a protective membrane referred to as the pleura. The lungs are also separated from the abdominal cavity by the muscular diaphragm.

Alveoli: These are tiny air sacs in the lung, where the actual exchange of gas (oxygen and carbon dioxide) occurs between the respiratory surfaces and the blood capillaries. There are about 480 million alveoli in the human lung. The alveoli are the final portion of the airway.

Pleural membranes: The pleurae are a doubled-layered serous membrane that surrounds the pleura cavity. The outer layer of the pleura is called the parietal pleura, while the inner layer is called the visceral layer. The parietal pleura attaches to the chest wall, while the visceral pleura surrounds the lungs, bronchi, blood vessels, and nerves. The main function of the pleural is to slow the full expansion and contraction of the lungs during breathing.

Pleura cavity: This is a fluid-filled space that surrounds the lungs. The pleural cavity is bounded by the pleura membrane. This cavity separates the lungs from surrounding structures such as the thoracic cage, mediastinum, diaphragm, and intercostal spaces.

The thorax: The thorax is located between the inferior region of the abdomen and the superior region of the root of the neck. The thorax forms the thoracic wall, breast tissues, and the thoracic cavity.

There are five muscles of the thoracic wall, which include the external intercostal, internal intercostal, innermost intercostal, subcostalis, and transversus thoracis.

The thoracic cavity contains organs and tissues that are important in respiration, digestion, cardiovascular, and nervous function.

The mediastinum: The mediastinum is located in the central compartment of the thoracic cavity between the pleural sac of the lungs. The mediastinum houses the heart and other important structures like the blood vessels, esophagus, thymus, and lymph nodes. Note that the mediastinum does not house the lung.

The diaphragm: This dome-shaped muscle is the major muscle involved in respiration. It is located just below the lungs and the heart. It contracts and flattens when you inhale and relaxes when you exhale.

Mechanism of Respiration

When you inhale, air passes through your windpipe and then through the bronchi to the alveoli at the ends of the bronchi. The alveoli are surrounded by capillaries (small blood vessels). Oxygen passes through the alveoli into the bloodstream. In the bloodstream, red blood cells pick up the oxygen and carry it to different body organs and tissues.

When the red blood cells release oxygen, they pick up carbon dioxide. The blood cells carry carbon dioxide back to the lungs and into the alveoli. When you exhale, carbon dioxide is expelled out of the bronchi through the trachea.

The Pulmonary Vascular System

In general, there are two types of circulation: systemic circulation and pulmonary circulation.

Systemic circulation involves the flow of blood from the heart to other parts of the body, while pulmonary circulation involves the flow of blood between the heart and lungs.

Pulmonary circulation is a network of arteries, veins, and lymphatics that exchange blood and other tissue fluids between the heart and lungs for oxygenation and back to the heart again. This system is important for ventilation and gas exchange.

Important components of the pulmonary vascular system include:

Arteries: Arteries carry blood away from the heart. The walls of the arteries are thicker than the walls of the vein because arteries experience more pressure as blood is pumped to the rest of the body. The walls of the arteries also have more smooth and elastic tissues than the vein.

Veins: Veins return blood to the heart. Veins have thinner and less elastic walls than arteries as the pressure pushing blood through them is not as much as those in arteries. Veins also have valves that help prevent the backflow of blood.

Capillaries: Capillaries are the smallest blood vessels in the vascular system. They deliver blood, oxygen, and nutrients to your organs and body system. They also connect branches of arteries to branches of veins.

Pulmonary arteries: The pulmonary arteries transport deoxygenated blood to the arterioles and capillaries beds in the lungs. Pulmonary arteries are the only arteries that carry deoxygenated blood.

Pulmonary veins: The pulmonary arteries carry oxygenated blood from the capillary bed into the left atrium of the heart. Pulmonary veins are the only veins that carry oxygenated blood. There are primarily four pulmonary veins.

Anatomy and Physiology of the Circulatory System

The Blood

Blood is a fluid connective tissue made up of 55% plasma, and the remaining 45% includes red blood cells, white blood cells, and platelets. It helps regulate the pH of body tissues, the water content of body cells and the chemical balance of the body.

Components of blood

There are four main components of blood: red blood cells, white blood cells, platelet, and plasma.

Red blood cells: The red blood cells (RBC) are also called erythrocytes. These cells are responsible for carrying oxygen and carbon dioxide between the lung and body tissue. These blood cells possess a compound called hemoglobin. Microscopically, the red blood cell appears as a biconcave disc.

Erythropoiesis is the process by which RBC is produced in the bone marrow. When the RBC matures, they are released into the bloodstream and last for 100-120 days. Anemia is a condition caused by a lack of red blood cells. Polycythemia, the opposite of anemia, is a condition in which there is an excess of red blood cells produced.

White blood cells: White blood cells (WBC), also called leukocytes, help the body to fight off infections and also assist in the immune process. The white blood cells lack hemoglobin and have a nucleus.

There are different types of WBC. These include lymphocytes, monocytes, eosinophils, basophils, and neutrophils.

The lymphocytes are further divided into two: the T lymphocytes and B lymphocytes. The B lymphocytes secrete antibodies that fight against foreign microorganisms. The T-cells help recognize and destroy virally infected and cancerous cells.

The monocytes and neutrophils are phagocytes. They help clean up debris from the site of infection. The eosinophils take part in allergic inflammatory reactions. They help destroy parasites that cause allergies. Basophils are also important in allergic inflammatory reactions. The bone marrow produces about 60-70% of the WBC; the rest is produced by the thymus, the spleen, and the lymph nodes.

The number of white blood cells fluctuates with activities. For example, there is a lower count of WBC during rest and higher values during exercise.

Platelets: Also called thrombocytes, platelets play an important part in wound healing. They help to control bleeding by forming blood clots. Platelets are shaped like plates.

Plasma: Plasma is the liquid component of the blood. The red blood cells, white blood cells, and platelets are suspended in the plasma.

The Heart

The heart is a muscular organ responsible for pumping blood to different parts of the body. It collects deoxygenated blood from all parts of the body to the lungs where it is oxygenated; in the process, it releases carbon dioxide. The heart then carries the oxygenated blood from the lungs to other parts of the body.

An adult heartbeat is about 60 to 80 beats per minute. The heartbeat of a newborn is much faster at about 70 to 190 beats per minute.

The heart is surrounded by a protective fluid sac called the pericardium. The walls of the heart consist of three layers: The epicardium (the outer layer), the myocardium (the middle layer) and the endocardium (the innermost layer).

There are four chambers in the heart. A partition, known as a septum, subdivides the heart into right and left halves. A constriction then divides each half into two cavities. The upper cavity is called an atrium, while the lower half is called the ventricle.

The right atrium: The right atrium receives deoxygenated blood from the body via the superior and inferior vena cava.

The left atrium: The pulmonary vein receives oxygenated blood from the lungs and drains it into the left atrium.

The right ventricle: The right ventricle is responsible for pumping blood to the lungs where it becomes oxygenated. The walls of the right ventricle are one-third less thick than the left.

The left ventricle: The left ventricle pumps blood to supply it to the body. It receives oxygenated blood from the left atrium and pumps it to the rest of the body. Because it takes more pressure to supply blood to the rest of the body than to the lungs, the walls of the left ventricle are three times thicker than those of the right.

The vena cava

The vena cava is the largest vein in the body. It has two parts: the superior vena cava and the inferior vena cava.

The superior vena cava carries blood from the upper extremities like the head, neck, arms, and chest to the heart.

The inferior vena cava carries blood from the lower limbs and organs in the abdomen to the heart. The inferior vena cava is found at the posterior abdominal wall, on the right side of the aorta.

The Cardiac Conduction System

The cardiac conduction system is a network of specialized cells found in the heart that control the heartbeat.

There are five major components of the cardiac conduction system.

1. The sinoatrial node (SA node):

The SA node is also referred to as the pacemaker of the heart. The SA node is the first component of the cardiac conduction system and sets the rate and rhythm of the heartbeat. SA nodes set the pace of the heart at 60-100 bpm.

The cells in the SA node are self-excitatory and can contract independently of an extrinsic innervation.

The SA node is responsible for generating electrical impulses/signals that cause the atria to contract. The signal then passes through the atrioventricular node to the ventricles.

The SA node is found in the atrial wall, between the superior cava vein and the right atrium.

2. The atrioventricular node (AV node)

The atrioventricular node is the second component of the cardiac conduction system. It is a small structure responsible for connecting the electrical systems of the atria and the ventricles. It transmits impulses into the ventricles.

The cells in the AV node are also self-excitatory, which makes it very useful in generating signals when the SA nodes are dysfunctional. When the SA nodes are unable to generate impulses, the AV nodes act as a secondary pacemaker, generating impedance from the atria to keep the ventricles contracting in their absence.

One important characteristic of the AV node is its ability to slightly delay an electrical impulse, so the atria contract first, before the ventricles.

3. Bundle of HIS

The bundle of His is a group of specialized muscle fibers that connect the atrial and ventricular chambers of the heart. They transmit impulses from the atrioventricular nodes to the bundle branches.

4. The bundle branches

The Bundle of HIS divides into two bundle branches, also known as the Tawara branches. The left bundle branch conducts impulses to the left ventricle, while the right bundle conducts impulses to the right ventricle. These bundle branches form into numerous smaller branches called Purkinje fibers.

5. Purkinje fibers

Purkinje fibers are branched fibers that carry impulses from the atrioventricular (AV) node to the ventricles causing them to contract and pump blood to the rest of the body. The Purkinje fibers are located in the inner ventricular walls of the heart.

The following is a summary of the occurrence of a heartbeat:

The SA node generates impulses causing the atria found in the upper chambers of the heart to contract. The signal then travels through the AV node, bundle of His, bundle branches and Purkinje fibers, causing the ventricles to contract. The SA fires another impulse and the circle begins. This normal sequential flow of electric impulses produces a normal heartbeat.

The Cardiac Cycle

The cardiac cycle is the series of events that starts from the beginning of one heartbeat to the beginning of the next. It involves the alternate contraction and relaxation of the atria and ventricles.

The cardiac cycle has two phases: the diastolic phase and the systolic phase.

The diastolic phase: In the diastolic phase, the heart is in a state of relaxation. In this stage, the heart chambers fill with blood through the vein.

The systolic phase: In the systolic phase, the heart chambers contract, and blood is ejected through the arteries.

Furthermore, the cardiac cycle can be divided into four stages:

- Filling phase: The ventricles fill with blood during diastole and atrial systole. At the end of the diastole, the atria contract, allowing a small amount of extra blood to enter the ventricles. This raises the pressure inside the ventricles.

- Isovolumetric contraction: The ventricles contract, increasing pressure and preparing to pump blood into the aorta/pulmonary trunk.

- Outflow phase: The ventricles continue to contract, pushing blood into the aorta and pulmonary trunk. This is also referred to as systole.

- Isovolumetric relaxation: The ventricles relax in preparation for the next filling phase.

Important terms to know about the cardiac cycle:

Cardiac output: Cardiac output (CO) is a measure of the amount of blood each ventricle pumps in one minute. To calculate cardiac output, stroke volume (SV) is multiplied with heart rate (HR).

Mathematically, CO is given as:

$CO = HR \times SV$

Stroke volume: Stroke volume is the volume of blood ejected out of the left ventricles during the systolic contraction. It is the difference between the end-diastolic volume and the end-systolic volume.

Mathematically it is written as:

$SV = EDV - ESV$

The normal range of SV in a 70kg (150lb) man is 50 to 100 ml. During exercise, the SV can increase to around 130 ml due to increased strength of contraction.

Factors affecting stroke volume:

- Heart size
- Gender
- Fitness levels
- Preload
- Afterload
- Duration of contraction
- Contractility

Heart rate (HR): This is the number of times the heart beats each minute. Adults have a normal resting heart rate of 60 to 100 beats per minute. During exercise, the HR in healthy young individuals can reach 150 beats per minute or higher. Factors affecting heart rate include:

- Age
- Fitness levels
- Certain hormones

Calculating estimated age-predicted maximum heart rate:

Example: What is the estimated age-predicted maximum heart rate of a 55-year-old female who is 6'1" tall and weighs 140 lbs. with a resting heart rate of 65 beats per minute?

The estimated maximum age-predicted heart rate would be calculated as 220 – age (years)= beats per minute (bpm).

So, for a 55-year-old:

Maximum heart rate = 220 - 55 = 165 beats per minute.

The individual's height, weight, and resting heart rate do not affect this calculation. However, keep in mind that the estimated age-predicted maximum heart rate is just that—an estimate.

Ejection fraction: This is the portion of the blood that is pumped out of the heart with each contraction. It takes into account both the amount of blood pumped out and the amount remaining in the ventricle.

The Karvonen Formula

The Karvonen formula is a mathematical equation used to calculate an individual's target heart rate training zone. It takes into account the person's maximum heart rate, resting heart rate, and desired training intensity to determine the target heart rate.

It is given as:

Target HR = ((max HR − resting HR) × %Intensity) + resting HR

Example:

What would be the target heart rate training zone for a 25-year-old with a resting heart rate of 65, who wants to work out at an intensity level of 60% to 70%?

Solution:

Step 1: Calculate the maximum heart rate (HRmax): HRmax = 220 - age

Step 2: Calculate the heart rate reserve (HRR): HRR = HRmax - resting heart rate

Step 3: Determine the desired intensity: For a target intensity of 60% to 70%, the desired intensity can be expressed as 0.6 × HRR to 0.7 × HRR

Step 4: Calculate the target heart rate: Target heart rate = resting heart rate + (desired intensity × HRR)

For a 25-year-old with a resting heart rate of 65:

HRmax = 220 - 25 = 195

HRR = 195 - 65 = 130

Desired intensity = 0.6 × 130 to 0.7 × 130 = 78 to 91

Target heart rate = 65 + 78 to 65 + 91 = 143 to 156

The target heart rate training zone for this individual would be between 143 and 156 beats per minute.

Blood Pressure

Blood pressure is a measure of the pressure within the large artery, or the force used to pump blood within the body. Blood pressure is measured using a sphygmomanometer and expressed in millimeters of mercury (mmHg) and is represented by two figures: the systolic and the diastolic pressure.

Blood pressure is often expressed in terms of the systolic over the diastolic pressure. For example, if a blood pressure reads 140 over 90, then it means the systolic pressure is 140, while the diastolic pressure is 90.

As a general guide:

- Normal blood pressure is considered to be between 90/60mmHg and 120/80mmHg

- Low blood pressure is considered to be below 90/60mmHg

- High blood pressure is considered to be 140/90mmHg or higher

Someone with blood pressure over 180/110mmHg is considered to be in a critical state. This stage is called a hypertensive emergency.

Physiological Adaptations to Exercise, Training, and the Impact of Recovery Strategies

Physiological Adaptation to Exercise and Training

Physiological adaptations are always specific to the type of training and amount of stress that the body is subjected to. These adaptations lead to an improvement in performance following training and are lost when training stops. These adaptations lead to better improvement when training involves various activities.

Some physiological adaptations that occur during training include:

- Decreased resting heart rate

- Increased stroke volume

- Increased cardiac output

- Increased oxygen uptake

- Increased hemoglobin levels in the blood

- Muscle hypertrophy

- Other changes in muscles like increased myoglobin and increased mitochondria

Decrease in resting heart rate

The normal resting heart rate for adults ranges from 60 to 100 beats per minute. However, training reduces heart rate. Some athletes have a resting heart rate of as low as 30-40 beats per minute.

One of the physiological adaptations that helps decrease the resting heart rate in athletes is an increase in stroke volume. Because there is an increase in the amount of blood pumped during each contraction, the heart will have a lower rate of contraction while transporting the same volume of blood.

Another physiological adaptation that decreases the resting heart rate in athletes is increased hemoglobin levels. Increased hemoglobin levels transport more oxygen per milliliter or liter of blood. In order to give the same amount of oxygen, the body needs to move less blood than a non-trained person.

These two adaptations increase oxygen transport, thus reducing cardiac contractions to meet basal metabolic oxygen needs. A decreased resting heart rate allows an athlete to increase their heart rate to its maximum and perform prescribed workloads at higher intensities and longer duration than an untrained athlete.

Increase in stroke volume and cardiac output

Stroke volume and cardiac output increase with training, increasing blood flow as a result. This increase in blood flow enhances oxygen delivery to functioning muscles. This increase in the amount of oxygen delivered delays fatigue by increasing aerobic training demands.

In addition, training leads to an increase in stroke volume, allowing the heart to pump the same amount of blood throughout the body with fewer contractions.

Increased stroke volume directly results in an increase in cardiac output since an athlete's maximum heart rate doesn't change much.

Increases in stroke volume and cardiac output are important physiological adaptations in athletes as they speed up blood and nutrient transfer, including oxygen. In turn, an athlete can remove lactate and carbon dioxide faster and give more oxygen and glucose to the muscle. Since lactate clearance and oxygen supply are faster, the athlete can train harder. In addition, because blood glucose and carbon dioxide are delivered faster, athletes can maintain these intensities longer.

Increase in oxygen uptake

Oxygen uptake increases in response to exercise, allowing for faster and more efficient oxygen delivery to the muscles. This increase in oxygen uptake increases the amount of oxygen transported into the blood for the muscle's use during aerobic activity.

The reason oxygen uptake increases during exercise and training is an increase in hemoglobin and myoglobin levels.

Aerobic exercise causes the body to produce more hemoglobin, which increases the oxygen-carrying capacity of the blood.

The increased use of aerobic energy systems delays the need for the body to employ anaerobic energy systems, thus preventing muscle exhaustion caused by acid buildup. Therefore, increasing hemoglobin levels increase the athlete's anaerobic threshold workload. This allows athletes to maintain higher intensities for longer because they stay in their aerobic training zone.

Muscular hypertrophy

Muscular hypertrophy is an increase in the cross-sectional area of the muscle caused by an increase in the number of myofibrils.

Muscular hypertrophy increases muscle strength and endurance. This increase in muscle cells improves athletes' performance by allowing them to use more force and repeat movements. In addition, hypertrophy increases muscular contraction speed, allowing for more power to be generated during contraction.

Muscle hypertrophy is beneficial in sports that demand strength, power, or muscular endurance, such as rugby, shot put, sprinting, football, ice hockey, and martial arts.

Effects on fast- and slow-twitch muscle fibers

Exercise and training have a wide range of effects on fast- and slow-twitch muscle fibers, depending on the type of training.

Adaptations in the fast-twitch muscle fibers lead to the use of anaerobic energy systems. Some of these adaptations include:

- Increased anaerobic enzymes for glycolysis
- Increased creatine phosphate stores
- Muscular hypertrophy
- Increased removal of lactate (this helps to reduce the acidic levels in the muscle)

Adaptations in the slow-twitch muscle fibers lead to the use of aerobic energy systems. Some of these adaptations include:

- Increase of mitochondria
- Increased capillary density
- Increased aerobic enzymes needed for ATP production
- Increased glycogen and fat stores, and myoglobin

Neural and Muscular Adaptations to Training Over Time

The rate of adaptation to strength and endurance training is influenced by various factors including intensity, volume, frequency, and initial fitness level.

People who have no prior training experience have the greatest adaptation potential and show rapid gains in strength or endurance.

Resistance training causes both neural and muscular adaptations, with neural changes happening faster. The improvement in strength initially seen in a resistance training program is mostly due to neural adaptations and improves as the central nervous system becomes better at muscle coordination and motor unit recruitment. Increases in muscle size also contribute to strength and can be seen within three weeks of starting a resistance training program.

Both neural and peripheral adaptations contribute to muscle force production, but muscle size determines the upper limit of strength. Cortisol has one of the most significant influences on neural changes.

Aerobic endurance training brings profound adaptations to skeletal muscle, increasing its ability to use oxygen for energy production and delaying fatigue during low-intensity contractions. The improvement in aerobic capacity depends on training intensity, with higher intensities leading to more rapid gains.

Impact of Recovery Stages

After competitions and training, people use recovery strategies to improve performance, adaptation, and wellness. A good recovery strategy also helps an athlete prevent injury and avoid overtraining.

One major importance of recovery is to continue training and performance at high intensities and for longer periods of time to further challenge the body and cause it to adapt. If, after competitions or training, recovery isn't observed, then the amount of training must be cut back. Otherwise, it can lead to overtraining.

There are four different types of recovery strategies: physiological, neural, tissue damage, and psychological strategies.

1. Physiological strategies

The aim of this strategy is to help the body recover from exercise physiologically. Some examples of physiological strategies include hydration and cool-down.

A cool-down after training or competition helps the body remove waste products and return back to its pre-exercise state. It helps speed up recovery by encouraging the continuous pump needed so that fluids move back to the heart, which helps in the removal of waste products. Examples of cool-down exercises include a light jog or a slow swim. However, the type of slow-down exercise used is specific to the type of sport and the major muscle used.

The second physiological strategy is hydration. Hydration involves drinking enough liquid like water or a sports drink after a competition to replace any fluid that was lost during the training or competition. Hydration helps to speed up recovery because dehydration can slow down or stop some recovery processes. It also adds more volume to the blood to aid the removal of waste products.

2. Neural strategies

This recovery strategy is focused on helping the nervous system recover. Some examples of neural strategies include hydrotherapy and massage.

Hydrotherapy involves water immersion. It is especially beneficial for sports that require a lot of muscle tension, such as football or rugby.

Hydrotherapy in warm water helps to relax the nervous system and the muscles it controls. In addition, they help the athlete relax and recover faster so that the athlete is ready to play again.

Massage is another recovery strategy that helps athletes to reduce tension and also relax their nerves. It helps to minimize the effects of fatigue, remove waste products, and reduce tension in the muscle. Some examples of massage include Swedish massage, myofascial, trigger point, and sports massage.

3. Tissue damage strategies

This strategy focuses on repairing damaged tissue, especially soft tissue, as well as any injury that happens from physical activity. This type of damage is often found in highly strenuous activities such as rugby. Some examples of tissue damage strategies include cryotherapy and compression garments and bandaging.

Cryotherapy involves using many forms of cold treatments like ice packs, cryogenic chambers, and cold water immersion to remove heat from damaged tissue and decrease inflammation and pain.

For soft tissue injuries, ice packs are placed over an athlete's injury to speed up recovery and should be used for 24 to 48 hours. This helps decrease inflammation, oxygen demand, and waste products.

For cryogenic chambers, athletes are placed in chambers at temperatures of around -110°C for a short time (usually less than three minutes). This helps to release endorphins, which relieve pain.

Ice baths are used for cold water immersion. The athlete is immersed in water that is set at a temperature of 4 to 12°C for 3-5 minutes at a time. The athlete is then brought out of the water before being resubmerged. This process is repeated four to five times.

Cold water immersion aids in reducing fluid buildup in the body caused by tissue damage. It also alleviates pain. However, using this technique repeatedly can impair performance.

4. Psychological Strategies

The focus of this strategy is on reviving the mind and creating a space for the athlete to relax. Some examples of psychological strategies include relaxation, sleep, debriefing, rest days, and sleep. Relaxation helps to decrease heart and respiration. It also helps to reduce nervousness in anxious patients.

<u>Metabolic Consequences of the Adaptations of Muscle to Endurance Exercise</u>

Some metabolic consequences of the adaptations of muscle to endurance exercise include:

- Slower utilization of muscle glycogen and blood glucose
- Greater reliance on fat oxidation
- Less lactate production during exercise
- Increase in the number and size of mitochondria
- Increase in capillaries and muscle blood flow

Special Consideration of Differences Among Athletes

<u>Athletes with disabilities</u>

Athletes with either congenital or acquired disabilities might develop conditions that affect their learning and development. Because children with congenital disabilities may not have the same opportunity to learn basic movement skills at the active start stage, parents and caregivers must have the information to help these athletes choose acceptable sports and activity programs.

In addition, some athletes with disabilities need personal assistance, interpreters, and other staff who may not be present in able-bodied sports. Athletes will suffer long-term if the sport system does not create these supporting positions.

Furthermore, many athletes with disabilities require modified facilities or adapted equipment to maximize their athletic potential and reduce potential disability-induced barriers.

<u>Age</u>

The decline in physiological function that occurs with aging is nearly identical to the decline in function that occurs with inactivity. In older adults, maximal heart rate and maximal stroke volume are reduced; thus, maximal cardiac output is reduced, resulting in oxygen levels lower than in a young adult. Thus, a coach must consider the athlete's age when designing a training, competition, and recovery program.

In sports, there are different types of ages to keep in mind. They include:

Chronological age: A measure of maturity or development based on the number of months or years that have passed.

Biological age: A measure of maturity determined by factors such as bone development, physical maturity, and sexual maturity.

Somatic age: This represents the extent of growth in overall height or specific parts of the body (such as limb length).

Training age: The period of time that a child has consistently engaged in a structured and supervised weightlifting program.

Gender: Being male or female does not affect an athlete's response to training. The response to training is based on individual willingness to train and genetic factors. However, due to some biological differences between genders, training should be more personalized.

For example, females cannot reach the muscle capacity of males because they have a lower level of testosterone. Females can benefit from weightlifting programs that are right for their age and build muscle strength and endurance. These programs may assist these athletes in improving their performance and limiting sport-related injuries.

The female's genetic potential and sports training allow competition in basketball, volleyball, swimming, and other sports. Due to their shorter extremities and lower center of gravity, adolescent females have an edge over their male counterparts in gymnastics and other balance sports.

Scientific Research and Statistics in the Exercise Sciences

The ability to effectively analyze and interpret data is very important when conducting and critiquing scientific literature. As professionals, it is important for exercise scientists to understand the basis of academic research as well as the statistical methods used to conduct that research.

When it comes to physiological studies, there are four techniques that are especially important. These include:

(1) Bivariate correlation and linear and non-linear regression

(2) Multiple regression

(3) Repeated-measures analysis of variance

(4) Multilevel modeling

The Applied Research Model for Sport Science is one proposed model that sports scientists can use when planning a study (ARMSS).

The ARMSS model uses both exploratory and experimental study designs that are linked together in a certain order to ensure that the research can be used in a sport setting as much as possible.

There are eight stages in the ARMSS model. These include:

- Defining the problem

- Descriptive research (hypothesis generating)

- Predictors of performance

- Experimental testing of predictors

- Determinants of key performance predictors

- Efficacy studies (controlled laboratory or field)

- Barriers to uptake

- Implementation studies (real sporting setting)

Sports Psychology

The Ideal Performance State is a highly focused state of mind where an athlete has confidence in their abilities and allows their performance to unfold effortlessly without any hindrances.

The three main objectives of sports psychology are:

1. Determining psychological aspects through measurement

2. Studying the relationship between psychological variables and athletic performance

3. Implementing theoretical knowledge to enhance athletic performance

Definitions of Key Concepts in Sports Psychology

Anxiety

- State anxiety: A current experience of worry and uncontrolled excitement.

- Trait anxiety: A personality trait that results in perceiving situations as a threat.

- Cognitive anxiety: Refers to mental processes and worrying thoughts.

- Somatic anxiety: Refers to physical symptoms like tense muscles, rapid heartbeat, and nervousness.

Stress: A disruption in mental and physical balance. Stress can be negative (distress) or positive (eustress).

Stressor: An event that triggers stress, whether it is environmental or cognitive in nature.

Attention and Skill

- Attention: The processing of internal and external cues that come to awareness.

- Skill: The ability to focus on task-relevant cues and manage distractions, which can be learned.

- Selective attention: Refers to the suppression of task-irrelevant stimuli and thoughts—considered an athlete's level of focus.

Cue utilization

- Low levels of arousal can result in both relevant and irrelevant cues being noticed, as well as poor concentration levels.

- Moderate levels of arousal result in increased focus and exclusion of task-irrelevant cues.

- Too high levels of arousal may result in missing task-relevant cues.

Attentional style

- Internal-external: Refers to an introspective or externally oriented perspective.

- Broad-narrow: Refers to an integrative (broad) or highly selective (narrow) orientation.

Psychological Foundations of Performance

There are four psychological factors of sports and exercise that most affect an athlete's performance. They include motivation, self-confidence, concentration, and emotional control.

Motivation

Intrinsic motivation: Intrinsic motivation is a person's inner drive to be good at something and have control over their actions. For example, an athlete may play a sport because they love it and have a desire to be successful.

Extrinsic motivation: Extrinsic motivation refers to motivation that comes from external sources or rewards, such as money, recognition, fame, or medals. This motivation is driven by external factors rather than internal factors such as enjoyment or personal satisfaction.

Achievement motivation: Achievement motivation is a person's desire to compete or compare themselves with others. Someone with high achievement motivation will likely be a better athlete because they have a strong desire to compete. A key component of achievement motivation is perceived competence.

Positive and Negative Reinforcement in Coaching

Positive reinforcement: Positive reinforcement is when a person's behavior is rewarded for making it more likely to reoccur in the future. For example, a coach may give an athlete praise, awards, or other rewards for good performance. Coaches should focus on positive reinforcement to help athletes focus on what they are doing correctly. Punishment should be used sparingly, as it may cause athletes to focus on their mistakes.

Negative reinforcement: Negative reinforcement is when a negative experience is removed to make a positive behavior more likely to happen in the future. For example, a coach may remove a punishment for a player if they perform well.

Influence of Arousal on Performance

Inverted-U theory: This theory states that arousal helps performance to a certain point, but if arousal goes beyond this point, it can alter performance.

Optimal functioning theory: Different people perform best at different levels of arousal.

Catastrophe theory: When arousal and anxiety increase at the same time, it can cause a sudden drop in performance.

Drive theory: An increase in an individual's arousal or state of anxiety leads to an increase in performance.

Reversal theory: The impact of arousal and anxiety on performance depends on their interpretation. For example, for one athlete, high arousal might be interpreted as excitement and a sign of preparedness for competition, while for another athlete, it might be perceived as unpleasant and reflect a lack of self-confidence.

Mental Skills

Mental imagery and hypnosis are mental skills used by athletes to help improve performance.

Mental imagery: This involves utilizing all senses to imagine yourself performing an athletic activity.

Hypnosis: This is a state where you become highly suggestible, and positive ideas about your athletic potential can be planted in your mind.

Both mental imagery and hypnosis can be effective tools for improving psychological arousal and changing behavior or performance.

Systematic desensitization: A combination of mental and physical techniques that help an athlete replace a fear response to various cues with a relaxed response.

Relaxation Techniques

Relaxation techniques are used to help people feel less tense and more able to concentrate on their performance. There are several techniques, including breathing exercises, progressive muscle relaxation, and autogenic training.

Breathing exercises: Here, the attention is on breathing to clear the mind and improve the ability to focus.

Progressive muscle relaxation: For this technique, the tensing and relaxing of different muscle groups is alternated to become more aware of physical tension and learn control.

Autogenic training: Here, the muscle relaxation cycle is replaced with a focus on feelings of warmth and heaviness in different parts of the body.

Motor Learning and Skill Acquisition Techniques

Motor Learning

Motor skills are tasks that demand voluntary control over joint and body segment movements to attain a goal.

Motor skills learning is the process of learning a skill in which the individual refines and automates the desired movements through practice and assimilation.

Stages of Motor Learning

There are different models used to describe the stages of motor learning. However, one of the most popular is the model proposed by Fitts and Posner in the late 1900s.

According to Fitts and Posner, there are three stages of motor learning:

Stage 1: Cognitive stage

In this stage, the individual focuses on what to do and how to do it. Here, movements are slow, inconsistent, and inefficient. Movement is also majorly done consciously. At this stage, the focus is also on the feedback received from the coach. Another name for this stage is the verbal-motor stage.

In the cognitive stage, there tend to be frequent errors, large gains, and a lack of consistency. The coach's duty at this stage is to provide feedback, not mechanical intervention.

Stage 2: Associative stage

This stage is also known as the motor stage. In this stage, the athlete has had an unspecified amount of practice and is beginning to show an improvement in performance. The athlete's movements in this stage are more fluid, reliable, and efficient. The focus is on skills refinement, as the basic fundamentals have been established. In addition, the athlete is now associating specific cues with resolving the motor problem at hand.

Furthermore, the athlete has fewer errors and is more consistent. Naturally, the variability of performance will decrease here. The learner puts in a lot of conscious effort, often focusing on body movements.

Stage 3: Autonomous stage

At the autonomous stage, the skill has become accurate, consistent, and largely automatic. The athlete can perform a task with little-to-no conscious thought. The athlete at this stage is a self-learner. They can detect errors in their performance and make appropriate adjustments. However, Fitts and Posner believe that not all athletes will reach this stage.

<u>Factors affecting Motor Learning</u>

- Verbal instructions
- Memory
- Postural control
- Practice distribution
- Practice variability
- Active participation and motivation
- Feedback
- Practice volume
- Practice difficulty
- Focus of attention

Motor Control

Motor control is defined as the ability to regulate mechanisms necessary for movement. There are six major theories of motor control described in practice. They include reflex theory, dynamic systems theory, hierarchical theories, motor program theory, ecological theory, and stimulus theory.

Reflex theory

According to this theory, reflexes are the basis for movement. Movement is controlled by stimulus-response. This theory relies heavily on feedback.

Dynamical systems theory

This theory proposes that movement emerges to control degrees of freedom. The authors of this theory believe that functional synergies emerge naturally as a result of practice and experience and aid in the problem of coordinating multiple muscles and joint movements simultaneously.

Hierarchical theories

According to this theory, cortical centers control movement throughout the nervous system from the top down. Furthermore, the theory postulates that voluntary movements are initiated by one's will and that reflexive movements take precedence only after CNS damage.

Motor program theory

This theory proposes the existence of adaptive, flexible motor programs (MPs) and generalized motor programs (GMPs) to control actions with similar characteristics.

Ecological theories

According to this theory, interactions between the individual, the task, and the environment influence motor behavior and learning. Perceptual information needed to control movement is derived through the interaction of a person with any given environment.

<u>Systems model</u>

This theory posits that several body systems overlap in order to trigger synergies for the generation of motions that are structured around functional purposes.

<u>Differences Between Motor Control and Motor Learning</u>

Motor control is concerned with how we control movement and generate useful coordinated responses. Motor learning, on the other hand, is concerned with how our control of movement changes as a result of practice and experience.

Indicators of Mental Health Issues in Athletes

Some indicators of mental health issues in athletes include:

- Athletic performance and anxiety
- Interpersonal issues with team/coaches
- Excess alcohol or drug intake
- Decreased interest in sports
- Drastic weight loss/gain
- Nonchalant attitude toward sporting results
- Pounding heart, sweating, shaking
- Frequent mood swings
- Suddenly quitting

- Self-isolation

- Extreme fatigue

- Excessive worry or fear

- Changes in eating habits such as increased hunger when anxious or lack of appetite when anxious

- Sleep disturbances, especially falling asleep

Causes of Mental Health Issues in Athletes

- Genetic predisposition to mental health issues

- Death of family members or loved ones

- Negative thought patterns

- An athlete's poor performance (injury or overtraining syndrome)

Nutrition

Athletes must consume enough calories to meet their energy requirements. If energy requirements are not met, the body will use fat and lean body tissue as fuel. This will result in a decrease in strength and endurance.

<u>Standard Nutritional Guidelines</u>

- Calorie guidelines and portion control suggestions for fruits, grains, proteins, and oils are provided based on age and sex for those who get less than 30 minutes of moderate physical activity daily.

- Athletes, or those with higher physical activity levels, should adjust these guidelines to fit their unique dietary needs.

- My Plate is an app that serves as a starting point for athletes to assess their diet. A diet that includes a variety of foods from each food group is likely to provide adequate amounts of all vitamins and minerals.

- A diet that includes a variety of foods from each food group is more likely to fulfill a person's need for macronutrients (carbohydrates, proteins, and fats) and micronutrients (vitamins and minerals).

- Excluding an entire food group from a diet can result in lacking specific nutrients. For example, athletes who avoid dairy may struggle to meet their calcium, potassium, and vitamin D requirements. Similarly, excluding all animal products and fish can result in inadequate vitamin B12 intake.

Important terms to know

Recommended Dietary Allowance (RDA): The average daily level of intake required to meet the nutrient requirements of nearly all healthy people.

Adequate Intake (AI): A level assumed to ensure nutritional adequacy when evidence is insufficient to develop an RDA.

The Estimated Average Requirement (EAR): This is the average daily intake of nutrients that is deemed sufficient to fulfill the needs of half of the healthy population within specific life stages and genders.

Tolerable Upper Intake Level (TUL): The maximum daily intake that is unlikely to have a negative impact on health.

Nutritional Factors Affecting Health and Performance

There are five major factors that affect nutritional needs. These include:

- Gut health: For people with a compromised digestive tract, it may be difficult to digest and absorb vital nutrients.

- Stage of life: As you get older, your nutritional needs change, and your digestive function may deteriorate. It is important to tailor the nutritional needs of individuals based on their age.

- Location: Nutritional needs often change based on where you live. For example, in the northern hemisphere, which includes places like Europe, Canada, and North America, Vitamin D is deficient. Hence, foods rich in Vitamin D and supplements containing vitamin D are recommended.

- Fitness: People who engage in intensive exercise lose certain nutrients, especially electrolytes through sweating. Hence, this should be considered when meal planning for such individuals.

- Medications: Various medications can increase your need for certain nutrients. Proton pump inhibitors (PPIs), for example, are known to increase the risk of vitamin and mineral deficiencies affecting vitamin B12, vitamin C, calcium, iron, and magnesium.

Nutritional Needs of Various Athletes

Nutrition can help athletes perform better. The best way to stay healthy is to maintain an active lifestyle and exercise routine, as well as to eat well. When athletes do not get enough nutrients, they are more likely to be tired and perform poorly during sports.

Nutritional needs in athletes include carbohydrates, proteins, fats, vitamins, minerals, and water.

Carbohydrates

Carbohydrates are required for energy during exercise. They are primarily stored in the muscles and liver. It is recommended that a little more than half of your calories should come from carbohydrates.

Carbohydrates can be broadly divided into two: simple sugars and complex carbohydrates.

Simple sugars include soft drinks, candy, and jellies. These foods contain "empty calories" because they contain a lot of carbohydrates but no vitamins, minerals, or other nutrients.

Foods containing complex carbohydrates include pasta, bagels, whole-grain breads, and rice. They supply energy as well as fiber, vitamins, and minerals.

Small amounts of carbohydrates (simple and complex) including carbohydrate-rich juice increase performance during sustained high-intensity sports lasting more than one hour.

Carbohydrates are needed for athletes planning to train for more than one hour. Immediate sources of energy include a glass of fruit juice, a cup of yogurt, or an English muffin. Limit fat intake in the hour before an athletic event.

Carbohydrates are also required during exercise if you plan to do more than an hour of intense aerobic exercise. This requirement can be met by having sports drinks, handfuls of pretzels, or low-fat granola bars.

As a general guideline, it is recommended that athletes consume approximately 30-60 grams of carbohydrates per hour before exercise.

Proteins

Protein is required for muscle growth and tissue repair. Protein can also be used as energy by the body, but only after carbohydrate stores have been depleted. According to the American Dietetic Association (ADA), adult athletes should consume 1.2 to 2.0 grams of protein per kilogram of body weight. In contrast, sedentary adults should consume 0.8 grams of protein per kilogram of body weight.

Despite popular belief, a high-protein diet does not promote muscle growth. This is a myth. Only strength training and exercise will result in changes in muscle mass.

People who do not consume enough protein in their daily diet may experience slower recovery and training adjustments. Taking amino acid supplements and consuming a lot of protein is not advised.

<u>Water and other fluids</u>

Water is the most important, yet often overlooked, nutrient for athletes. Your body requires water and fluids to stay hydrated and at the proper temperature. One hour of vigorous exercise can cause your body to sweat several liters.

Drink plenty of fluids with each meal, whether or not you intend to exercise. It is important to begin exercising with enough water in your body. Drink about 16-20 ounces of water two hours before a workout. Continue to sip water during and after your exercise.

When exercising, water is best for the first hour of activity. You can switch to an energy drink after the first hour to help you get enough electrolytes. Clear urine indicates that you have fully rehydrated.

<u>Fats</u>

Fat is the primary fuel source for light-to-moderate intensity exercise. Fat is also a valuable metabolic fuel for muscles during endurance exercise, but it does not provide the quick bursts of energy required for speed.

Some sources of fat in foods include:

- Dairy products such as cheese, whole milk, sour cream, and ice cream
- Cooked meats and fish

- Nuts or avocados

- Processed foods such as chips, crackers, granola bars, and French fries

Athletes should consume 20-35% of their total daily calories as fat. Current dietary guidelines recommend that 10% of fat intake come from monounsaturated sources, 10% from polyunsaturated sources, and no more than 10% from saturated fat.

<u>Vitamins and minerals</u>

Vitamins and minerals play an important role in optimizing the health of athletes. They take part in the prevention of oxidative damage, blood synthesis, energy production, tissue, and muscle repair during recovery from exercise or injury, maintenance of bone health, and immune function.

Vitamins are divided into two: Fat-soluble vitamins and water-soluble vitamins.

Fat-soluble vitamins include vitamins A, D, E, and K. Vitamin B and C are water-soluble vitamins.

Fat-soluble vitamins can become toxic when consumed in high amounts, as these vitamins accumulate in the body. Vitamin A toxicity, also known as hypervitaminosis A, can occur from consuming large amounts of preformed vitamin A from animal-derived sources such as liver and cod liver oil, or from taking high-dose vitamin A supplements.

Water-soluble vitamins, on the other hand, are generally considered safe in excess, as any excess is excreted by the body and not stored in the liver.

Important vitamins athletes should include in their diet are calcium, iron, zinc, magnesium, vitamin B, and vitamin D, as well as antioxidants like vitamins C and E, beta-carotene, and selenium.

Athletes who are vegetarian may not get enough iron, calcium, vitamin D, riboflavin, zinc, or vitamin B12. To compensate for these deficiencies, it's best to talk to a sports dietitian.

Health Risk Factors Associated with Dietary Choices

Overweight and obesity

Diets high in fat and calories are strongly linked to obesity. If you consume excessive amounts of energy, especially fats and sugars, and do not expend the energy through exercise and physical activity, the body will store much of the excess energy as fat.

Heart disease and stroke

High blood pressure and high cholesterol are two of the leading causes of heart disease and stroke. Excess sodium consumption can raise blood pressure and increase the risk of heart disease and stroke. Current guidelines recommend no more than 2,300 mg per day.

Eating foods high in fiber and low in saturated fat, as well as increasing access to low-sodium foods, can help prevent high blood cholesterol and high blood pressure.

Type 2 diabetes (T2DM)

Poor dietary habits and a sedentary lifestyle are the main causes of the increasing cases of diabetes mellitus in developing countries. A high-fat, high-calorie, and high-cholesterol diet increases the risk of diabetes. Consumption of red meat, sweets, and fried foods increases the risk of insulin resistance and T2DM.

Consumption of fruits and vegetables, on the other hand, may protect against the development of T2DM because they are high in nutrients, fiber, and antioxidants, which act as a protective barrier against the disease.

Eating Disorders

Eating disorders are a group of mental health disorders characterized by abnormal patterns of eating and weight control. They include anorexia nervosa, binge eating disorder, bulimia nervosa, avoidant/restrictive food intake disorder, pica, and rumination disorder.

Anorexia nervosa: This eating disorder is characterized by severe restriction of food intake, leading to dangerously low body weight, intense fear of gaining weight, and a distorted body image.

Binge eating disorder: This is characterized by recurrent episodes of binge eating. Individuals who binge eat consume large amounts of food in a short period of time and feel a lack of control over the behavior.

Bulimia nervosa: This eating disorder is characterized by binge eating followed by purging behaviors, such as self-induced vomiting, fasting, or excessive exercise to eliminate calories consumed.

Avoidant/restrictive food intake disorder (ARFID): This is an eating disorder characterized by a refusal or avoidance of food that results in significant weight loss, malnutrition, or developmental delays in children.

Pica: Pica is an eating disorder in which an individual craves and eats non-food items, such as paper, chalk, or dirt.

Rumination disorder: Rumination disorder is a condition where a person regurgitates partially digested food and either re-chews, re-swallows, or discards it.

These disorders have a range of symptoms, including malnutrition, weight loss, digestive problems, and electrolyte imbalances.

It is important for athletes and their support teams to be aware of the symptoms of these disorders and to seek professional help when needed.

Note that the strength and conditioning professional is not responsible for treating eating disorders but should refer athletes to appropriate medical or mental health professionals.

Macronutrient calculations

In summary:

Carbohydrates (for every 1 g of carb = 4 calories (kcal))

Protein (1 g protein = 4 calories (kcal))

Fats (1 g fat = 9 calories (kcal))

Alcohol (1 g alcohol = 7 calories (kcal))

Sample calculation 1:

How many calories will a protein bar have if the protein bar has the following macros?

- Protein: 30 grams
- Carbs: 8 grams
- Fat: 2.5 grams

Protein 30 g x 4 calories = 120 calories

Carbs 8 g x 4 calories = 32 calories

Fat 2.5 g x 9 calories = 22.5 calories

120+32+22.5 = 174.5 calories

Calculating a calorie deficit to lose 1 lb of fat

To lose 1 lb of fat, an athlete needs to reduce their daily calorie intake by 3500 calories over a certain period.

To calculate a calorie deficit, you must first determine the athlete's TDEE, or Total Daily Energy Expenditure, which is their average energy usage per day.

Once you have this information, you can subtract their average calorie intake from their TDEE to find the deficit amount.

Mathematically,

Calorie Deficit= TDEE — Average calorie intake

For example, if an athlete wants to lose 3 lbs, they need a (3 × 3500) = 10, 500 calorie deficit, which can be achieved by eating 3,200 calories per day (a 300 calorie deficit per day) for 35 days, if they are very diligent in sticking to their calorie goals.

10,500 total calories / 300 calories per day = 35 days

Calculating protein requirement in sports

To calculate protein recommendations for athletes, you need to first determine their body weight in kilograms. This can be done by dividing their weight in pounds by 2.2.

For endurance athletes, the recommended protein intake is between 1.0-1.6 grams per kg of body weight.

For athletes that focus on strength it is between 1.4-1.7 grams per kg of body weight. If an athlete is aiming for weight loss or muscle gain, their protein intake can be increased beyond these ranges.

Note that the RDA of 0.8 grams per kg of body weight per day is not sufficient for athletes to optimize muscle protein synthesis.

Cunningham equation

The Cunningham equation helps coaches determine an athlete's resting metabolic rate (RMR), which provides an estimate of their total daily energy expenditure.

The basal metabolic rate (BMR) and RMR are different. The BMR is the energy needed for basic body and brain function without any additional demands from being awake, eating, or physical activity, and it must be measured in a fasted state.

On the other hand, RMR doesn't require fasting and includes the energy needed for food digestion.

The Cunningham equation can be used to calculate your resting metabolic rate.

The Cunningham equation is given as:

RMR = 500+22 × {kg of free fat mass}

Example 1:

If you have a 180 lb. male athlete, he would be approximately 81.8 kg. (180 / 2.2).

Next, you need to determine the % of body fat. If this athlete is 18% body fat you would take 81.8 kg x 0.18% = 14.72.

81.8-14.72 = 67.08 kg lean mass

500 + (22 x 67.08 kg) = RMR of 1975.76 calories

Example 2:

A 250 lb. male athlete has 5% body fat—0.05 equals 5% body fat.

First convert the weight to kg. To do this, divide the weight in lbs. by 2.2 to get the weight in kilograms.

250/2.2 = 113.63 kg

Then take the fat percentage and multiply it by the mass in kg.; this will give you the fat mass (FM)

113.63 x 0.05 = 5.68 kg

Next, calculate the fat-free mass (FFM). To do this, subtract the fat mass (FM) from the total weight in kilograms.

113.63 − 5.68 = 107.95 kg

Finally, use the Cunningham equation

RMR =500 + [22 x (FFM)]

RMR=500 + [22 x 107.95]

RMR=500 + 2374.9

RMR=2874.9 calories

Calculating the total calories needed from carbohydrates

A 300 lb. athlete has a 4000 daily kilocalorie intake and would like carbohydrates to represent 60% of this total. How many grams of carbohydrates must he consume per day?

Solution

First calculate the total number of kilocalories of carbohydrates that the athlete consumes based on his desired carbohydrate intake as a percentage of his daily kilocalorie intake.

Total daily kilocalories from carbohydrates = 60% of 4000 kilocalories/day = 0.6 x 4000 kilocalories/day = 2400 kilocalories/day.

Now convert the number of kilocalories from carbohydrates to grams of carbohydrates.

One gram of carbohydrates = 4 kilocalories.

So. the grams of carbohydrates the athlete should consume per day are as follows:

Grams of carbohydrates per day = Total daily kilocalories from carbohydrates / 4

Grams of carbohydrates per day= 2400 kilocalories/day / 4 = 600 grams/day.

Therefore, the athlete should consume 600 grams of carbohydrates per day.

Effects of Hydration Status and Electrolyte Balance/Imbalance on Health and Performance

Electrolytes are required for functions including hydration, muscle contraction, and blood pressure stabilization. Certain electrolytes, such as sodium and potassium, are lost through sweat and must be replaced to maintain proper fluid balance in the body. In addition, electrolytes aid in fluid absorption during exercise.

During exercise, the antidiuretic hormone (ADH) and the renin-angiotensin-aldosterone system maintain electrolyte and water homeostasis.

An imbalance of electrolytes in the body may lead to fatigue, dehydration, cramping, weakness, tingling, or confusion. Severe electrolyte imbalances can result in serious complications such as coma, seizures, and cardiac arrest.

The four most important electrolytes for athletes are sodium, magnesium, calcium, and potassium.

Sodium

Sodium aids fluid retention as well as nerve and muscle function, blood volume control, and blood pressure control.

Although this rarely happens, as many individuals meet and exceed their daily sodium recommendation, a lack of sodium will cause blood pressure to drop, leading to dehydration.

The daily sodium recommendation is 2300 milligrams per day. However, if you're an athlete who loses a lot of sodium through sweat, consuming more than 2300 milligrams per day is unlikely to cause any problems.

You can get more sodium in your meal by adding foods to your diet such as pickles, olives, pretzels, table salt, or saltine crackers.

Calcium

Calcium is important for bone health. It helps with nerve signaling, muscle contraction, blood clotting, hormone secretion, and normal heart function. Without enough calcium intake, the body draws calcium from the bones, causing them to weaken over time.

The daily calcium recommendation is 1000 milligrams per day.

You can get more calcium in your diet by consuming food such as dairy (milk, yogurt, cottage cheese, cheese), dried figs, chia seeds, leafy greens, soy products, fortified oatmeal, and more.

Magnesium

Magnesium relaxes the muscles and allows them to absorb oxygen. Additionally, it aids in the maintenance of a normal heartbeat and muscle function.

The recommended dietary allowance (RDA) for adults aged 19-to-51 years is 400-420 mg daily for men and 310-320 mg daily for women.

You can increase your magnesium intake by including the following foods in your diet: spinach, chard, edamame/soy, quinoa, beans, lentils, salmon, and nuts and seeds, such as pumpkin seeds, flax seeds, cashews, and chia seeds.

Potassium

Potassium is very important in hydration and muscle contraction. It also plays a major role in proper heart function.

Potassium deficiency can cause muscle weakness, cramping, and abnormal heart rhythms.

The daily potassium recommendation is 3500-4700 milligrams per day.

You can increase your potassium intake by including the following foods in your diet: bananas, dairy, oranges, winter squash, potatoes, broccoli, lentils, halibut, salmon, and apricots.

Effects, Risks, and Alternatives of Common Supplements

Vitamin D

Vitamin D increases calcium absorption in the body and helps to prevent bone diseases such as osteoporosis.

Many athletes take vitamin D supplements because getting enough from food is difficult. Vitamin D blood levels above 100 nanograms per milliliter, on the other hand, can cause extra calcium absorption, which can result in muscle pain, mood disorders, abdominal pain, and kidney stones. It may also increase the risk of having a heart attack or a stroke.

You can increase vitamin D intake by spending 10 to 15 minutes per day in the sun without sunscreen.

Antioxidants (vitamin C, vitamin E, and coenzyme Q10)

Antioxidants such as vitamin C, vitamin E, and coenzyme Q10 help to reduce free-radical damage to skeletal muscle, resulting in less fatigue, inflammation, and soreness.

High doses of vitamin C (more than 2,000 mg/day in adults) can cause diarrhea, nausea, abdominal cramps, and other gastrointestinal problems.

In adults, taking more than 1,500 IU/day (natural form) or 1,100 IU/day (synthetic form) of vitamin E increases the risk of hemorrhagic effects.

Excess coenzyme Q10 consumption may result in nausea, heartburn, and other side effects.

Arginine

Arginine increases blood flow and oxygen and nutrient delivery to skeletal muscle. It also acts as a substrate for creatine production and stimulates muscle growth by increasing human growth hormone secretion.

Reported adverse effects include nausea, abdominal pain, diarrhea, bloating, gout, headache, allergic response, airway inflammation, or worsening of asthma symptoms.

Beta-alanine

Beta-alanine increases the synthesis of carnosine, thereby reducing muscle fatigue. It also enhances performance by increasing exercise capacity.

Reported adverse effects include paresthesia (tingling in the face, neck, back of hands, and upper trunk) and pruritus (itchy skin).

Beta-hydroxy-beta-methylbutyrate (HMB)

Beta-hydroxy-beta-methylbutyrate aids in the repair of damaged skeletal muscle cells. It also improves exercise adaptations, reduces muscle loss, and promotes faster recovery after exercise.

HMB supplementation at three grams per day appears well tolerated and is not associated with any negative side effects. However, in rare cases, people taking HMB may experience stomach pain, constipation, or itching.

Betaine

Betaine is a popular bodybuilding supplement. It increases hydration, stimulates water-based pumps, boosts power, and promotes protein synthesis. Betaine can also help with endurance and resistance training.

Betaine supplementation has no known serious side effects. However, in some people, it can cause nausea, upset stomach, and diarrhea.

Citrulline

Citrulline dilates blood vessels, increasing oxygen and nutrient delivery to skeletal muscle. It also helps to widen your blood vessels (vasodilation) and may help with muscle building.

There are no reported side effects of L-citrulline. However, some people might experience stomach discomfort.

Creatine

Creatine provides energy to muscles for short-term, mostly anaerobic activity. It may also help to improve athletic performance and increase muscle mass.

Reported adverse effects of creatinine include weight gain due to water retention, muscle strains and pulls, nausea, diarrhea, muscle cramps, muscle stiffness, and heat intolerance.

Quercetin

Quercetin increases the number of mitochondria in muscles, lowers oxidative stress, reduces inflammation, and improves blood flow. Quercetin also boosts antioxidant activity and promotes muscle growth.

Quercetin is widely regarded as safe. Headaches and upset stomach are possible side effects.

Iron

Iron increases oxygen uptake, lowers heart rate, and lowers lactate concentrations during exercise.

At doses greater than 45 mg/day, common side effects of iron include gastric upset, constipation, nausea, abdominal pain, vomiting, and fainting. Experts recommend taking supplements or eating high-iron meals in the morning, within 30-60 minutes of finishing a workout.

Performance-Enhancing Substances and Methods

Performance-enhancing substances (PEDs) are substances that are used to improve any type of activity performance in humans. People take performance enhancers to help during high-intensity physical activity.

Athletic performance-enhancing substances are sometimes referred to as ergogenic aids.

Performance-enhancing drugs can range from caffeine and sports drinks to illegal substances.

Common performance-enhancing substances include:

Anabolic steroids

Anabolic steroids are made from testosterone. They prevent muscle breakdown and preserve muscle mass. Most athletes use this substance to enhance performance.

Anabolic steroids work by mimicking the body's natural male hormone, testosterone, to help build muscle tissue and increase body mass.

Steroid use has been prohibited in the United States since the Anabolic Steroids Control Act of 1990. Anabolic steroids were banned in sports because they could give an athlete an unfair advantage over other competitors.

Some of the most common types of anabolic steroids include: stanozolol, nandrolone, boldenone, trenbolone, androstenedione, and tetrahydrogestrinone.

In general, potential side effects of these steroids include muscle hypertrophy, acne, increased blood pressure, thrombosis, altered libido, and male pattern baldness.

Females who use anabolic steroids may experience facial hair growth, amenorrhea (absence of menstruation), breast atrophy, and thickening of vocal cords (voice deepening).

Stimulants

Stimulants are substances used to increase focus and alertness. They also improve mental and physical performance by increasing muscle strength and endurance while decreasing reaction time and fatigue.

Stimulants are commonly used in long-duration exercises that necessitate short bursts of energy (e.g., tennis, team sports, etc.). Caffeine, ephedrine, cocaine, methylphenidate, and amphetamine are all examples of stimulants.

Hypertension, insomnia, headaches, weight loss, increased heart rate, tremors, anxiety, addiction, and strokes are all potential side effects.

Caffeine and other stimulants are legal and widely available in competitive sports. Other substances, however, such as cocaine, amphetamines, and ephedrine, have been prohibited by the World Anti-Doping Agency (WADA).

Human growth hormone (hGH)

hGH is one of the most commonly used substances among professional athletes because it has a small window for detection. Human growth hormone is banned in competition by the World Anti-Doping Agency. It is not permitted at any time or for any level of athlete, including elite, junior, and master athletes.

Potential side effects of hGH include cardiomyopathy, diabetes, renal failure, and hepatitis.

Blood boosters

Also known as blood dopers, it is an illegal method of enhancing athletic performance by artificially increasing the ability of the blood to deliver more oxygen to muscles.

Blood doping agents increase the oxygen-carrying capacity of blood beyond the natural capacity of the individual.

Blood dopers are used in endurance sports such as long-distance running, cycling, and skiing. Blood doping is prohibited by the International Olympic Committee and other sports organizations.

The three most common types of blood doping include:

- Blood transfusions

- Erythropoietin (EPO) injections

- Synthetic oxygen carriers

One of the most well-known drugs in this class is erythropoietin (EPO). Erythropoietin, or EPO, is a hormone that aids in the production of red blood cells, which improves oxygen delivery to muscles.

Potential side effects of erythropoietin include dehydration and an increase in blood viscosity, which could lead to a pulmonary embolism or stroke.

Diuretics

Athletes use diuretics as a masking agent to avoid the detection of another banned substance.

Diuretics are prohibited by the World Anti-Doping Agency. Diuretics increase the rate at which the body excretes water (which dilutes the urine) and alter how drugs are metabolized. Diuretics are prohibited because both actions have an impact on anti-doping tests.

In addition to masking other drugs, diuretics can help athletes lose weight, which they can use to their advantage in sports where they must qualify in a specific weight category.

Examples of commonly used diuretics by athletes include furosemide, bendroflumethiazide, and metolazone.

Insulin

Insulin promotes glucose uptake into the muscle and aids in the formation and storage of glycogen in the muscle. Athletes use insulin for events that require high levels of endurance.

Bodybuilders use insulin in conjunction with anabolic steroids such as testosterone or human growth hormone to build muscle tissue. Steroids create new muscles, and insulin prevents them from breaking down.

Insulin also improves stamina in middle-distance runners and other track athletes by allowing them to load their muscles with glycogen "fuel" before and between events.

Insulin abuse or overdose can result in low blood sugar levels, a condition known as hypoglycemia, which can cause cognitive function loss, seizures, unconsciousness, and, in extreme cases, brain damage and death because the brain is starved of energy and oxygen.

<u>Beta-blockers</u>

Beta-blockers inhibit sympathetic effects, such as increases in heart rate and blood pressure, which are often increased during athletic competition.

Beta-blockers are prohibited in certain sports that rely on the stability of the extremities, such as archery, racing, darts, billiards, and pistol shooting, because they are thought to unfairly improve a user's skills.

Common beta-blockers used include carvedilol, metoprolol, atenolol, and propranolol.

Impact of Alcohol and Drugs on Performance

Acute alcohol use can have an impact on motor skills, hydration status, aerobic performance, and other aspects of the recovery process. When you consume alcohol, your blood alcohol concentration rises. After this, the acute side effects begin, which can lead to depression of the central nervous system.

The effects of alcohol vary depending on the dose, and they can result in impaired motor skills, decreased coordination, delayed reactions, impaired judgment, and impaired balance.

Even small amounts of alcohol consumed prior to exercise can reduce endurance performance. Alcohol impairs aerobic performance by slowing the citric acid cycle, inhibiting gluconeogenesis, and raising lactate levels.

Chronic alcohol use can result in nutritional deficiencies and lowered immune function, increasing the risk of injury, and requiring more time to heal. Many nutrients are affected by alcohol absorption and utilization. Excessive alcohol consumption can impair the ability of the intestine to absorb nutrients such as vitamin B12, thiamine (B1), and folate. Furthermore, liver cells can become inefficient at activating vitamin D, and alcohol metabolism can destroy vitamin B6.

Effects of Performance-Enhancing Drugs on Performance

<u>Physiological</u>

- Liver damage

- Male pattern baldness

- Breasts growth

- Lower levels of the "good" cholesterol

- High blood pressure

- Problems with the heart and blood flow

- Decrease in the size of testicles

- Dehydration

- Arrhythmias

- Myocardial infarction

- Stroke

- Seizures

- Risk of diseases such as HIV or hepatitis, if using needles to give shots of drugs

Psychological

- Increased aggressiveness and sexual appetite

- Issues with anger or violence

- Significant mood swings

- Depression

- Withdrawal symptoms such as headaches, anxiety, anorexia, depression, apathy

Chapter 3: Practical and applications

Exercise Technique

Exercise technique refers to the proper way to perform an exercise in order to achieve the desired results while minimizing the risk of injury. These techniques can differ depending on the type of exercise and the specific muscle groups targeted.

Examples of exercise techniques include a proper form for weightlifting, correct breathing patterns during cardio exercise, and proper alignment during yoga poses.

<u>Factors that affect exercise techniques</u>

- Differences in body type

- Muscular strength

- Power output

- Endurance

- Flexibility

- Motor/skill learning capabilities

- Other factors that can affect the exercise techniques used include injuries and medical conditions.

<u>Fundamentals of Exercise Techniques</u>

The basics of resistance training exercise techniques have several key elements common to most exercises. These include using a grip on equipment such as bars, dumbbells, or handles for free weight or machine exercises.

Other important elements in exercise technique are maintaining an ideal body or limb position, controlling movement range and speed, and proper breathing. Certain exercises may also require the use of a weight belt and specific procedures for starting the lift.

Hand grips

Two common grips in resistance training exercises are:

• Pronated grip: Palms down, knuckles up.

• Supinated grip: Palms up, knuckles down.

A variation of either grip is the neutral grip. The neutral grip is neither supinated nor pronated; instead, the palms are facing each other, and the knuckles are pointing forwards.

Other types of grips include:

• Alternated grip: One hand pronated, one supinated

• Hook grip: This is similar to the pronated grip, but with the thumb under the index and middle fingers. It is often used for power exercises and recommended for people with a weak grip.

Proper grip placement involves positioning hands at the correct distance from each other and from the center of the bar for balance.

There are three common grip widths: common, wide, and narrow. For most exercises, hands are placed approximately shoulder-width apart for a balanced bar.

There are two types of grips used in weightlifting exercises and their variations:

- The clean grip: This grip is in a pronated and closed-hand position. The clean grip is slightly wider than shoulder-width apart and outside of the knees.

- The snatch grip: This grip is also in a pronated and closed-hand position.

However, the snatch grip is a wide grip, determined by either the fist-to-opposite-shoulder method or the elbow-to-elbow method.

Stable body and limb positioning

Establishing stability during exercises, whether lifting a barbell or dumbbell from the floor or using machines, is important for safety and improved performance. A stable position allows the athlete to maintain proper body alignment and place appropriate stress on muscles and joints.

During standing exercises, feet should be positioned slightly wider than hip-width with both heels and balls of feet in contact with the floor. On machines, stability may be achieved by adjusting the seat or resistance arm and securely fastening belts.

The five-point body contact position

Exercises performed while seated or lying face up (supine) on a bench require proper posture. The athlete should position their body so that there are five points of contact with the bench.

1. The head is securely positioned on the bench or back cushion.

2. The shoulders and upper back are firmly and evenly supported by the bench or back cushion.

3. The buttocks are evenly positioned on the bench or seat.

4. The right foot is resting flat on the ground.

5. The left foot is resting flat on the ground.

Breathing considerations

For most resistance training exercises, athletes should exhale during the most strenuous phase of the repetition, known as the sticking point, and inhale during the less demanding phase.

The Valsalva maneuver, which involves exhaling against a closed glottis to increase rigidity of the torso and support the vertebral column, can be used by experienced athletes during high-load structural exercises. However, it is important that the athlete not hold their breath for too long, as this can cause potential side effects like dizziness, high blood pressure, and blackouts.

For most exercises, athletes should be asked to exhale through the sticking point of the concentric phase and inhale during the eccentric phase.

Weight belts

Wearing a weight belt can help maintain intra-abdominal pressure and reduce the risk of lower back injury during lifting.

It is best to wear a weight belt during exercises that stress the lower back and during sets with heavy loads.

However, excessive use of a weight belt can reduce abdominal muscle training and is not necessary for exercises that do not stress the lower back ((e.g., biceps curl, lat pulldown) or those that stress the back but with light loads (e.g., back squat or deadlift).

Free weight exercises

Most free weight exercises require a spotter. A spotter is someone who helps athletes perform exercises while ensuring their safety. This includes preventing injury and potentially assisting with forced repetitions. However, the primary responsibility of a spotter is to ensure the safety of the athlete.

Free weight exercises performed with a bar or dumbbells over the head, on the back, or on the front, such as barbell shoulder press, back squat, front squat, bench press, and lying triceps extension, are more challenging to execute correctly and require one or more spotters. These exercises, especially with dumbbells, are also potentially more dangerous and require more skill from the spotter.

Overhead exercises and those involving the bar on the back or front shoulders should be performed inside a power rack with crossbars in place and with all equipment cleared from the lifting area. The spotter should be at least as strong and tall as the athlete and should have a wide base of support. In addition, when spotting over-the-face exercises, such as the bench press or shoulder press, the spotter should stand behind the lifter.

The spotter should use an alternated grip and be positioned close to the bar or dumbbell when spotting over-the-face exercises. Spotting is not advised for power exercises, and athletes should be instructed on how to get away from an unmanageable bar.

When spotting dumbbell exercises, it is crucial to spot close to the dumbbells or, in some cases, to spot the dumbbell itself. Some people suggest spotting by placing their hands on the athlete's upper arms or elbows, but this method can be dangerous and cause injury. This is because if the athlete's elbows bend, the spotter won't be able to prevent the dumbbells from hitting the athlete's face or chest. Spotting near the athlete's wrists at their forearms is a safer technique. For specific exercises, such as the dumbbell pullover and overhead dumbbell triceps extension, it is necessary to spot using the hands on the dumbbell.

The number of spotters needed depends on the load being lifted and the experience and ability of the athlete and spotters.

How to perform exercises correctly

Lower body pushing: Lower body pushing exercises include exercises that work the muscles in the legs and glutes, such as squats, lunges, leg presses, and calf raises. To perform these exercises, you will need to use weightlifting equipment or your own body weight.

How to perform lower body pushing exercises

1. Squats: Stand with your feet shoulder-width apart and lower your body as if you were sitting back into a chair. Keep your chest up and your back straight as you lower your body. Push through your heels to return to the starting position.

2. Forward lunges: Step forward with one foot, bending both knees to lower your body. Keep your front knee directly above your ankle and your back knee close to the ground. Push through your front heel to return to the starting position.

3. Leg press: Sit in a leg press machine with your feet on the platform. Push the platform away from you, straightening your legs. Slowly lower the platform back to the starting position.

4. Glute bridges: Lie on your back with your knees bent and your feet flat on the floor. Your arms should be at your sides with your palms facing down. Drive your heels into the floor and raise your hips toward the ceiling. Keep your core engaged and your glutes contracted as you lift. Hold the position at the top for a moment, squeezing your glutes, then slowly lower your hips back down to the starting position. Repeat for the desired number of repetitions.

5. High-bar Olympic squats: This is also known as the "Olympic squat" or "high-bar back squat." The Olympic squat targets the quadriceps, glutes, and lower back muscles. It is a more advanced variation of the traditional back squat and is typically performed with a barbell and a squat rack.

Here are the steps to perform a high-bar Olympic squat:

- Set the barbell on the squat rack at about chest height.

- Position yourself under the barbell so that it sits on top of your upper back, just below the base of your neck.

- Grasp the barbell with a narrow, overhand grip, and lift it off the rack.

- Take a step away from the rack and set your feet shoulder-width apart, with your toes pointing slightly outward.

- Bend your knees and hips, lowering your body as if you were sitting back into a chair. Keep your chest up and your back straight as you lower your body.

- Continue lowering your body until your thighs are parallel to the ground, or slightly below parallel.

- Push through your heels to return to the starting position, straightening your legs and hips.

- Repeat for the desired number of reps, then carefully rack the barbell on the squat rack.

Deadlift

The deadlift is a compound exercise that works the back, hips, and legs muscles. It's usually done with a barbell, but it can also be done with dumbbells or kettlebells.

The deadlift is an excellent way to increase overall strength and muscle mass.

Here are the steps to perform a deadlift:

- Stand in front of a loaded barbell with your feet hip-width apart. Your toes should be pointing forward.

- Bend down and grip the barbell with an overhand grip, with your hands just outside of your legs.

- Keep your back straight and your chest up as you lift the barbell off the ground by straightening your hips and legs.

- As the barbell passes your knees, drive your hips forward and stand up fully.

- Lower the barbell back to the ground by bending your hips and legs, keeping your back straight and your chest up.

- Repeat the movement for the desired number of reps.

It's also important to remember that you should use a squat rack or a spotter when performing this exercise, as the weight can be quite heavy.

Sumo deadlift: The sumo deadlift is a variation of the traditional deadlift that targets the same muscle groups (back, hips, and legs muscles), but with a different stance and grip. The sumo deadlift is named after the sumo wrestling stance, characterized by a wide stance and a grip inside the legs.

Here are the steps to perform a sumo deadlift:

- Stand in front of a loaded barbell with your feet wider than hip-width apart, toes pointing outwards.

- Bend down and grip the barbell with a mixed grip, with one hand overhand and the other hand underhand, and with your hands inside of your legs.

- Keep your back straight and your chest up as you lift the barbell off the ground by straightening your hips and legs.

- As the barbell passes your knees, drive your hips forward and stand up fully.

- Lower the barbell back to the ground by bending your hips and legs, keeping your back straight and your chest up.

- Repeat the movement for the desired number of reps.

<u>Upper body pushing</u>

Upper body pushing exercises include exercises that work the muscles in the chest, shoulders, and triceps, such as the bench press, shoulder press, push-ups, and dips. To perform these exercises, you will need to use weightlifting equipment or your own body weight.

Types of upper body pushing:

1. Bench press: Lie on a flat bench with a barbell above you. Grasp the barbell with a slightly wider than shoulder-width grip. Lower the barbell to your chest and press it back up to the starting position.

2. Shoulder press: Sit on a bench with a barbell at shoulder height. Grasp the barbell with a slightly wider than shoulder-width grip. Press the barbell overhead, then lower it back down to the starting position.

3. Push-ups: Get into a plank position, with your hands placed slightly wider than shoulder-width apart and your body in a straight line. Lower your body by bending your elbows, and then press back up to the starting position.

4. Dips: Use parallel bars or the edge of a bench to perform dips. Lower your body by bending your elbows, and then press back up to the starting position.

5. Barbell flat bench press: The barbell flat bench press is a compound exercise that targets the chest, shoulders, and triceps. It is typically performed with a barbell and a weight bench.

<u>Here are the steps to perform a barbell flat bench press:</u>

- Lie on a flat-weight bench with your eyes under the barbell.

- Grasp the barbell with a slightly wider than shoulder-width grip, with your palms facing forward.

- Unrack the barbell by lifting it off the supports and bringing it straight over your chest.

- Lower the barbell to your chest by bending your elbows, keeping your wrists straight.

- Push the barbell back up to the starting position by straightening your arms, keeping your elbows tucked in close to your body.

- Repeat the movement for the desired number of reps.

6. Standing overhead press: The standing overhead press, also known as the "shoulder press," targets the shoulders, triceps, and upper back muscles. It is typically performed with a barbell but can also be done with dumbbells or kettlebells.

<u>Here are the steps to perform a standing overhead press:</u>

- Stand with your feet shoulder-width apart and hold a barbell at shoulder level with a grip that is slightly wider than shoulder width.

- Keep your core engaged and press the barbell overhead by extending your arms straight up.

- Lower the barbell back to your shoulders by bending your elbows.

- Repeat the movement for the desired number of reps.

Upper body pulling

Upper body pulling exercises include exercises that work the muscles in the back, biceps, and forearms, such as pull-ups, chin-ups, rows, and lat pull-downs. To perform these exercises, you will need to use weightlifting equipment or your own body weight.

- Pull-ups: Hang from a pull-up bar with an overhand grip, slightly wider than shoulder-width. Pull your body up toward the bar, keeping your elbows close to your body. Lower yourself back down to the starting position.

- Chin-ups: Hang from a pull-up bar with an underhand grip, slightly narrower than shoulder-width. Pull your body up toward the bar, keeping your elbows close to your body. Lower yourself back down to the starting position.

- Rows: Sit at a rowing machine or use a barbell or dumbbells. Hold the weight(s) with an overhand grip and pull the weight(s) toward your chest, keeping your elbows close to your body. Lower the weight(s) back down to the starting position.

- Lat pull-downs: Sit at a lat pull-down machine and grasp the bar with an overhand grip, slightly wider than shoulder-width. Pull the bar down toward your chest, keeping your elbows close to your body. Release the bar back to the starting position.

Weightlifting (Olympic lifting movements)

Weightlifting is a sport that consists of two lifts: The snatch and the clean and jerk. These movements, which are usually performed with a barbell, necessitate a high level of skill, strength, and technique.

1. Snatch:

- Stand in front of a barbell with your feet hip-width apart.

- Bend down and grasp the barbell with a wide, overhand grip.

- Lift the barbell off the ground by extending your hips and knees.

- As the barbell reaches your hips, quickly pull yourself under the bar by dropping into a squat and catching the barbell in an overhead squat position.

2. Clean and jerk:

- Stand in front of a barbell with your feet hip-width apart.

- Bend down and grasp the barbell with a wide, overhand grip.

- Lift the barbell off the ground by extending your hips and knees.

- As the barbell reaches your hips, quickly pull yourself under the bar by dropping into a squat and catching the barbell on your shoulders (front squat position).

- Stand up with the barbell and then press it overhead by extending your arms (jerk).

Before we proceed, here are some essential terms you should know:

Agonist: An agonist muscle is a muscle that is primarily responsible for producing a specific movement. This muscle contracts and generates force to produce the movement. It's also referred to as the prime mover muscle. For example, in a bicep curl, the agonist muscle is the bicep muscle. It's the muscle that is actively contracting and causing the arm to move.

Antagonist: This is the opposite of the prime mover. The antagonist muscle helps to control or stabilize the movement produced by the agonist muscle. For example, in a bicep curl, the antagonist muscle is the triceps. It works to keep the elbow steady and control the movement of the arm as the bicep contracts.

Synergist: The synergist muscle is also known as the helper muscle. This muscle supports the agonist muscle and helps it to perform the movement more efficiently. In exercise, a synergist muscle is a muscle that works in conjunction with the agonist muscle to produce a specific movement.

For example, in a bicep curl, the agonist's muscle is the bicep muscle that contracts to lift the weight, and the synergist muscle is the brachioradialis muscle, which is located in the forearm. It helps to stabilize the elbow joint and assists the bicep in lifting the weight.

Stabilizer: Stabilizer muscles are muscles that work to maintain proper posture and control movement during an exercise and help to prevent injury and improve overall muscle balance and stability. They are also referred to as fixator muscles or neutralizer muscles.

For example, during a barbell squat, the quadriceps and glutes are the agonist muscles that contract to lift the weight, but the muscles of the core, such as the transverse abdominus, internal oblique, and rectus abdominis are stabilizer muscles that help to maintain proper alignment and stability of the spine, pelvis, and hips.

Movement Preparation

Movement preparation, also known as a dynamic warm-up, involves movement in different directions and at different speeds to help activate the tissues as well as the nervous, circulatory, and respiratory systems, which are in charge of controlling and fueling movement.

Fundamental movements

There are seven basic movements, also known as functional movement patterns, that the human body can perform. All other exercises can be classified as variations of these seven basic movement patterns. These movements include:

Pull: Exercises that involve pulling a weight toward the body, such as pull-ups and rows. These movements primarily target the mid and upper back, biceps, forearms, and rear shoulders. Examples of pull exercises include lat pulldown, bent-over row, and biceps curls.

Push: This is the opposite of the pull. Push exercises involve pushing a weight away from the body, such as push-ups and bench presses. These exercises work the muscles in the chest, triceps, and front shoulders. Examples of push exercises include bench presses, shoulder presses, triceps extensions and more.

Squat: This involves exercises that involve sitting back and down, such as squats and lunges. The squat targets the glutes, core, quadriceps, and to an extent, the hamstring muscles.

Rotation: These exercises involve rotating the core, such as Russian twists and wood chops. Rotation exercises are used to target the muscles of the core, including the abs, obliques, and lower back.

Hinge: This involves exercises that involve bending at the hips, such as deadlifts and good mornings. Hinge exercises are used to target the muscles of the posterior chain, including the glutes, hamstrings, and lower back.

Lunge: Exercises that involve stepping forward with one foot and lowering the body, such as lunges and step-ups. This movement requires greater flexibility, stability, and balance. Like squats, the lunge targets the glutes, quadriceps, core, and hamstrings. However, the split stance stimulates all three gluteal muscles to a greater extent than squats.

Gait: Exercises that involve movement of the body in a linear direction, such as walking and running. These exercises are essential for improving overall cardiovascular fitness, endurance, and functional movement.

Movement preparation exercises

Movement preparation exercises, also known as dynamic stretching or warm-up exercises, are exercises used to prepare the body for movement prior to a workout or physical activity. They are used to increase flexibility and range of motion, as well as to activate muscles that will be used during the workout.

Keep in mind that movement preparation exercises should be done before your workout and should be tailored to the athlete's specific workout.

Here are some examples of movement preparation exercises:

- Lunges
- Arm circles
- Inchworm
- Leg swings
- High knees
- Jumping jacks
- Thoracic rotation

Resistance Training Exercise Technique

Resistance training involves exercises that use external resistance to increase muscle strength, tone, mass, and endurance. The resistance can be provided by various objects such as dumbbells, exercise tubing, or even the person's own body weight.

Resistance training works by causing damage to muscle cells, which prompts the body to repair and strengthen the muscles, resulting in increased muscle growth.

There are several styles of resistance exercise. They include:

(1) Olympic lifting

(2) powerlifting

(3) weightlifting

Benefits of Resistance Exercise

- Increases muscle strength and tone
- Reverses the effects of aging by building muscle mass
- Strengthens bones
- Boosts metabolism and helps maintain body weight.

Effects of Resistance Exercise

A. Muscle hypertrophy

Higher training volumes are linked to increased hypertrophy (muscle size). This is achieved through a moderate-to-high number of reps per set (6 to 12) and 3 to 6 sets per exercise. The most effective strategy for increasing muscle size is to perform three or more exercises per muscle group. These training volume assignments can lead to substantial gains.

B. Muscle endurance

Resistance training programs aimed at increasing muscular endurance typically involve performing 12 or more reps per set with lighter weights and fewer sets, usually 2 or 3 per exercise. This results in a lower overall volume-load.

C. Strength and power

The recommended range for strength training is two-to-five or three-to-six sets for core exercises and only one-to-three sets for assistance exercises. The volume for power training is lower to maximize the quality of exercise and typically involves three-to-five sets after a warm-up.

Resistance Training Techniques

Common techniques include:

1. Progressive overload:

Progressive overload is the practice of gradually increasing the weight or resistance used in exercises over time to make gains in muscle size, strength, and endurance. To achieve this, one can increase weight, reps, sets, or manipulate rest periods. It is an important principle in strength training as the body adapts to the demands placed on it, so in order to continue making progress, the demands must be increased over time.

Progressive overload can be achieved by:

- Gradually increasing the weight, reps, and sets

- Decreasing rest time

- Adding resistance bands, chains, or other equipment

- Varying exercises

- Increasing the frequency or duration of the workout.

Each of these methods places additional stress on the muscles, helping to continue progress and adaptations.

One of the major drawbacks of progressive overload training is that it has to be done gradually. If the load or frequency of your training is increased too quickly, it can lead to injury.

2. Repetition ranges

Repetition ranges refer to the number of times a specific exercise should be performed in a set. For example, a repetition range of 8-12 means a person should perform the exercise 8-12 times in a set. Different repetition ranges are associated with different training goals. For example, low repetition ranges (1-5) and heavy weights are used for building muscle mass and strength, while high repetition ranges (12-15 or more) with lighter weights are used for muscular endurance.

In addition, repetition ranges are also associated with different muscle fiber types. Low repetition ranges (1-5 reps) are associated with fast-twitch muscle fibers, and high repetition ranges (12-15 or more) are associated with slow-twitch muscle fibers.

3. Tempo

In weightlifting, tempo refers to the speed at which you lift and lower the weight during exercises, known as the concentric and eccentric phases of movement, respectively. This is usually represented by a 3- or 4-digit number, with each number indicating the pace at which a particular portion of the exercise should be done.

In strength training, tempo refers to the speed at which an exercise is performed. It is often represented by a 4-digit number, such as 3-0-1-0, that indicates the length of time (in seconds) spent during each phase of the exercise: the eccentric (lowering) phase, the pause at the bottom, the concentric (lifting) phase, and the pause at the top.

For example, a tempo of 3-0-1-0 would indicate that the eccentric phase should last three seconds, and there should be no pause at the bottom; the concentric phase should last 1 second, and no pause at the top.

Different tempos can be used to achieve different training goals. A slower tempo can help increase muscle activation and time under tension, while a faster tempo can help increase power and explosiveness.

4. Rest periods

This simply means taking a specific amount of time to rest between sets. In strength training, rest periods refer to the time taken between sets of an exercise.

The length of the rest period can vary depending on the exercise, the individual's goals, the number of reps, and the weight used. For example, 1-2 minutes of rest is used for exercises with heavy weights and low reps to allow muscle recovery, while shorter rest periods of 30-60 seconds are used for exercises with lighter weights and higher reps to increase muscle endurance.

Rest periods can also be used to manipulate exercise difficulty and play a role in determining the overall volume of a workout.

5. Supersets and giant sets

In strength training, a superset is a method of performing two exercises back-to-back without rest, typically for different muscle groups.

A giant set, also known as a compound set, is similar to a superset but involves performing two or more different exercises back-to-back for the same muscle group.

6. Drop sets

A drop set is a method used in strength training where an individual performs a set of an exercise to fatigue, then immediately reduces the weight and continues to perform more reps with the lighter weight. This process is repeated one or more times, with the weight being dropped each time until the individual can no longer perform the exercise with proper form.

Drop sets are used to increase muscle fatigue, push the muscle to failure, and lead to increased muscle hypertrophy. They can also be used to increase muscle endurance and target specific muscle fibers.

7. Isolation exercises

Isolation exercises are exercises that are specifically designed to target a single muscle or muscle group. Examples of isolation exercises include bicep curls, tricep extensions, leg extensions, and calf raises. These exercises can be useful for addressing specific areas of weakness or for creating muscle definition.

8. Compound exercises

Compound exercises are those that engage multiple muscle groups at once. Furthermore, these exercises typically use more than one joint, which can improve overall mobility and stability. Examples of compound exercises include squats, deadlifts, bench presses, rows, pull-ups, and dips. These exercises are highly effective for developing overall muscle mass and strength, as well as enhancing functional fitness.

In addition, compound exercises tend to burn more calories than isolation exercises, making them a great option for weight loss or weight management.

Repetition Maximum (RM)

A Repetition Maximum (RM) measures the heaviest weight an individual can lift for a specific number of repetitions with proper technique.

For example, a 10RM would be the heaviest weight a person could lift for ten consecutive reps. It is a standard method used by strength and conditioning coaches to evaluate an individual's current strength level, identify strength imbalances, and measure the effectiveness of training programs.

By determining and tracking 1RM, it is possible to monitor an individual's progress and make adjustments to their training program as needed.

1RM can be determined directly through maximal testing or indirectly through submaximal estimation methods, such as the Brzycki formula.

The Brzycki formula is given as:

(weight / (1.0278 − 0.0278 × reps).

For example, if you just managed to lift 50 kg for five reps, you'd calculate your 1RM like this:

50 / (1.0278 - 0.0278 × 5) = 56.25 kg

The type of muscle development achieved depends on the specific combination of reps, sets, exercises, resistance, and force. Generally, the RM (Repetition Maximum) range can be used as a guide:

- For muscle power development, 1-6 RM per set should be used and performed explosively.

- For muscle strength and power development, 3-12 RM per set should be used, with fast or controlled movements.

- For muscle strength and size development, 6-20 RM per set should be used, with controlled movements.

- For muscle endurance development, 15-20 or more RM per set should be used, with controlled movements.

When conducting a 1RM test, it is crucial to select the right exercises that can accurately assess strength while ensuring the athlete maintains proper form. Estimating an athlete's 1RM can be done using prediction equations or a 1RM table. The training load and repetition assignments should be based on the athlete's training goal, which can be determined using the repetition maximum continuum or a percentage of the 1RM.

To increase the training load over time, the 2-for-2 rule is a conservative method to be used to increase an athlete's training load, which involves adding weight to the exercise if the athlete can perform two or more repetitions over their assigned repetition goal in the last set in two consecutive workouts. The quantity of load increases can be varied based on the athlete's size, strength, and training status, with a smaller, weaker, and less trained athlete requiring a smaller load increase than a larger, stronger, and more trained athlete.

Calculations

To calculate the weight that should be used when using a resistance band, we need to subtract the resistance provided by the band from the total resistance needed to lift for the 10RM.

Weight with resistance band = Total resistance — Resistance provided by the band

Olympic Weightlifting and Plyometric Exercise Technique

Olympic weightlifting

The main exercises in Olympic weightlifting are the clean and jerk, snatch, and variations of these two exercises.

The snatch is an Olympic lift consisting of four fundamental components executed as a single fluid lift. Proper training and technique can help anyone master the snatch lift. The lift starts with a setup, followed by a pull, and ends with the bar above the head and the body motionless. High-hang snatches can help build explosiveness and increase the speed of getting under the bar.

The snatch requires pulling the bar up with the muscles in the legs, back, and glutes, and lifting it above the head by getting under the bar in a squat position.

The clean and jerk involves pulling the bar high, clearing the shoulders, and thrusting the weights overhead under control using the triple extension of knees, ankles, and hips. The lift then transitions to a frontal squat before jerking the bar overhead.

These two movements can create a lot of power at the hips, which can translate to an explosive hip extension when sprinting, jumping, or changing direction. Olympic weightlifting often involves lifting heavy loads. One major disadvantage of Olympic lifting is that it requires a significant amount of coaching time and attention, and there is limited variety in the movement patterns.

Plyometric exercises

Plyometric exercises involve quick and powerful movements using a pre-stretch or countermovement, utilizing the stretch-shortening cycle (SSC). These exercises typically require minimal to no load, unlike Olympic weightlifting, which often involves much heavier loads.

Plyometric training is often considered to be the link between strength and performance.

Models of plyometric exercise

There are two models of plyometric exercise: the mechanical model and the neurophysiological model.

- Mechanical model

The mechanical model of plyometric exercise explains how the elastic energy in the muscle and tendons is increased through a rapid stretch and then stored.

This stored energy is later released during a subsequent concentric muscle action, resulting in an increase in total force production.

The series elastic component (SEC), which is primarily made up of tendons, plays a crucial role in plyometric exercise.

The SEC acts as a spring and stores energy during an eccentric muscle action and releases this energy during a concentric muscle action. If a concentric muscle action does not immediately follow the eccentric action, the stored energy will be lost as heat.

- Neurophysiological model

The neurophysiological model in plyometric exercise involves the potentiation of the concentric muscle action through the stretch reflex, which is the body's involuntary response to a quick stretch of the muscles.

The reflexive component of plyometric exercise is primarily composed of muscle spindle activity, which increases muscular activity in response to a rapid stretch. This reflexive response increases the force produced by the muscle, but if there is too much time between the stretch and the concentric muscle action, the potentiating ability of the stretch reflex is lost.

The stretch-shortening cycle

Plyometric exercises utilize the stretch-shortening cycle (SSC), which is a lengthening movement followed by a shortening movement.

The SSC is a process that enhances muscle recruitment by utilizing the energy storage capabilities of the musculotendinous system (SEC) and the stretch reflex.

There are three phases of the SSC cycle:

- Eccentric phase: Involves the preloading of the agonist muscle group.

- Amortization phase: This phase entails the delay between the eccentric and concentric muscle actions.

- Concentric phase: This phase details the body's response to eccentric and amortization phases.

Mode of plyometric exercise

Plyometric training involves exercises that target either the upper or lower body, depending on the body region performing the exercise.

Lower body plyometrics are suitable for various sports, such as track and field, soccer, volleyball, basketball, and endurance sports, as they require the athlete to produce a maximum amount of force in a short time.

Some examples of lower body plyometric drills are:

- Jumps in place
- Standing jumps
- Multiple hops
- Bounds
- Box drills
- Depth jumps (this is considered to be the most intense plyometric drills)

Upper body plyometrics, on the other hand, are important for sports that require rapid and powerful upper body movements, such as baseball, softball, tennis, and golf.

The upper body plyometric drills include:

- Medicine ball throws
- Catches
- Push-ups

Note: Athletes weighing over 220 pounds may be more susceptible to injury during plyometric exercises due to the increased compressive force on joints. To reduce injury risk, these athletes should avoid high-volume, high-intensity plyometric exercises and depth jumps from heights higher than 18 inches.

Equipment and Facilities for Plyometric Exercise

• The landing surface for lower body plyometrics should be shock-absorbing and appropriate surfaces include grass fields, suspended floors, or rubber mats.

• Concrete, tile, and hardwood floors are not recommended due to their lack of shock-absorbing properties.

• Thick exercise mats and mini trampolines are not effective for plyometric training of uninjured athletes because they extend the amortization phase.

• The amount of space required for plyometric drills varies based on the type of drill being performed. Bounding and running drills typically need at least 30 meters of straightaway space.

• For standing, box, and depth jumps, only a small surface area is needed, but the ceiling height must be between three to four meters.

• Boxes used for box jumps and depth jumps should be sturdy, have a nonslip top and a height range between 6 and 42 inches, and have landing surfaces of at least 18 by 24 inches

• Participants should wear footwear with good ankle and foot support, lateral stability, and a wide, non-slip sole.

• The recommended height for depth jumps ranges from 16 to 42 inches, with 30 to 32 inches being the norm.

- For athletes who weigh over 220 pounds, the height of the depth jump box should be 18 inches or less.

Speed/Sprint Technique and Agility Technique

Speed and sprint techniques refer to the proper form and mechanics used when running at high speeds.

Sprinting technique training can be divided into five categories: starting, acceleration, drive phase, recovery phase, and deceleration.

Speed, change of direction, and agility are key components of athletic performance.

- Speed is the ability to reach maximum velocity and acceleration.

- Change of direction refers to the physical capacity to change direction during activity.

- Agility involves a combination of physical and cognitive abilities to change direction in response to a stimulus.

Speed and Agility Mechanics

The force an athlete generates in executing movement techniques is a product of mass and acceleration.

Mathematically, Force= Mass (M) × Acceleration (A)

There are two variables that describe force: rate of force development (RFD) and impulse.

RFD is the development of maximal force in minimal time and is an index of explosive strength.

Impulse is the product of the generated force and time and determines the magnitude of momentum change.

Physics of sprinting, change of direction, and agility

Speed is the rate of an object's movement, while velocity is speed with direction.

Acceleration is the rate at which an object's velocity changes.

The ability to generate force rapidly is desirable in sports, with RFD being a more useful measure than maximal force production. To achieve higher acceleration, an athlete should apply forces at a greater rate.

Impulse is the product of the time a force is applied and the amount of force applied. It results in changes in momentum and can be represented as the area under a force-time curve.

Impulse is important in sprinting and change of direction, as it influences the ability to accelerate or decelerate. The only way to increase impulse is to generate greater force.

The production of braking forces over a period of time, known as braking impulse, is also important in change of direction and agility. The time constraint in agility can limit the time available to produce the required impulse, making it physically more demanding to perform.

For sprinting to be successful, training should focus on impulse and rate of force production (RFD).

Momentum is defined as the relationship between mass and velocity.

Sprint speed

Sprint speed is a combination of stride length and stride rate. A successful sprinter is one who has a longer stride length as a result of applying more force into the ground and a more frequent stride rate.

The amount of vertical force applied to the ground during the stance phase is considered the most critical component of improving speed.

Elite sprinters are able to achieve higher velocities through high-force application during a short stance phase, resulting in longer strides occurring at a higher rate.

The limiting factors for sprint speed include rapid force production (RFD), technical efficiency, and proper training.

Sprinting technique

The linear sprinting technique is divided into three stages: the start, acceleration, and top speed. These stages require the athlete to move their lower limbs at maximum speed through stance and flight phases.

The start phase is further broken down into eccentric braking and concentric propulsive periods, while the flight phase consists of recovery and ground preparation.

The start of the sprint requires balanced body weight distribution, aggressive extension, and a high horizontal velocity.

During acceleration, the recovery of the swing leg should be low to the ground, and elite male sprinters display a stride rate of 5.26 steps/second and stride length of 1.13-1.15 m during the first two steps of block clearance.

Maximum velocity requires the SSC to propel the center of mass horizontally. The fundamental training objectives include brief ground support times and the development of the SSC to increase impulse.

Key variables to monitor in sprinting

- Step length
- Stride Length
- Flight time
- Stride Angle
- Speed
- Acceleration

Key variables to monitor in agility

- Change-of- direction deficit
- Ground contact time
- Exit velocity
- Entry velocity
- Decision Making Time

Fundamental movements in maximum-velocity sprinting

1. Early flight

- Eccentric hip flexion decelerates the backward rotation of the thigh.
- Eccentric knee extension decelerates the backward rotation of the leg/foot.

2. Mid-flight

- Concentric hip flexion accelerates the thigh forward.
- Eccentric knee extension to eccentric knee flexion.

3. Late flight

- Concentric hip extension rotates the thigh backward in preparation for foot contact.
- Eccentric knee flexion accelerates the leg backward, limiting knee extension and preparing for foot contact, aided by concentric knee flexion.

4. Early support

- Concentric hip extension minimizes the braking effect of foot strike.
- Brief concentric knee flexion followed by eccentric hip extension: resists knee hyperextension during landing and absorbs shock.
- Eccentric plantarflexion: helps absorb shock and control the forward rotation of the tibia over the ankle.

5. Late support

- Eccentric hip flexion decelerates the backward rotation of the thigh.
- Concentric knee extension propels the center of gravity forward.
- Concentric plantarflexion aids in propulsion.

<u>Common errors in sprinting technique</u>

- Hips being too high at the start of the crouch position
- Stepping out laterally during the initial drive phase

- Abnormally short and tight arm movement

- Unnecessary tension in the dorsal muscles

- Jumping the first stride or stepping over the knee of the stance leg

Here are some speed drills you can try:

- A-skip

- Fast feet

- Sprint resistance

Here are some agility drills you can try:

- Deceleration drill

- Agility drill (Y-shaped agility)

- Z-drill

- 5-10-5 shuttle

Energy Systems Development

Energy System Development (ESD) is a training method that aims to increase the efficiency of the body's energy systems to improve athletic performance. It involves training the three main energy systems used by the body during physical activity. These include the phosphagen system, the glycolytic system, and the oxidative system.

The three energy systems include the phosphagen system, the glycolytic system, and the oxidative system.

- The phosphagen system

The phosphagen system provides energy for short, high-intensity activities, such as weightlifting and sprinting. It uses stored creatine phosphate and adenosine triphosphate (ATP) to generate energy quickly.

- The glycolytic system

The glycolytic system provides energy for moderate-intensity activities that last up to 2 minutes, such as middle-distance running and high-intensity interval training. It uses glycogen stored in the muscles and liver to generate energy.

- The Oxidative System

The oxidative system provides energy for low-intensity activities that last for an extended period, such as endurance running and cycling. It uses fat and carbohydrate as fuel and generates energy through cellular respiration.

Recovery Techniques

Recovery methods for athletes include various techniques used to alleviate muscle soreness, fatigue, and injury after physical activity or competition. These may include hydrotherapy, active recovery, stretching, compression garments, massage, sleep, and a balanced diet with adequate protein, carbohydrates, and healthy fats. Keep in mind that recovery techniques may vary depending on the individual needs.

Some common recovery techniques used by athletes include:

- Stretching

- Massage therapy

- Active recovery (low-intensity activities like walking, swimming, or cycling)

- Ice therapy

- Hydrotherapy
- Eating a balanced diet
- Adequate sleep

Program Design

<u>Conducting Needs Analysis</u>

The needs analysis involves identifying the essential characteristics required for the athlete, the sport, or a combination of both.

Conducting a comprehensive needs analysis enables the strength and conditioning coach or sports scientist to determine the crucial physical attributes for their athlete to excel in their sport. It also provides an analysis of the sport's injury risks, which helps the coach to design training programs that can help prevent such injuries.

In general, needs analysis is conducted in three parts:

- Sport-orientated needs analysis
- Athlete-oriented analysis
- Comparative analysis

1. Sport-Oriented Needs Analysis

The first step in a needs analysis for sports is to identify the unique characteristics of that sport in order to design a specific training program. This can be done through the following analysis.

This type of analysis includes sports analysis, injuries analysis, biomechanical injuries, and physiological analysis to determine strength, power, and endurance priorities.

In addition, characteristics such as cardiovascular endurance, speed, agility, and flexibility should also be assessed.

Sports analysis: This analysis involves answering questions about the type of sport involved, the type of equipment to be used, the competition level (professional or amateur), the duration of the sport, and any other sports regulations, like if there are any rest times and what position the athlete plays.

Injuries analysis: This analysis involves finding out the common injuries in that sport and position, how frequently these injuries occur, predisposing factors to these injuries, and total injuries every year.

Biomechanical analysis: Biomechanics is divided into the areas of kinematics and kinetics. These analyses include identifying optimal techniques for enhancing sports performance, assessing muscle recruitment and loading, and analyzing the sport and exercise equipment, like shoes, surfaces, and rackets.

Aerobic and anaerobic analysis: This analysis includes analyzing average heart rate, VO2 max, maximum rate, lactate threshold, anaerobic capacity, and high intensity.

2. Athlete-oriented analysis

The second part of the needs analysis involves assessing the athlete's needs and goals through tests and evaluations to determine the best approach for the training program. The assessment process should be individualized to design specific programs for each individual, considering factors such as current condition, previous injuries, and exercise history.

This analysis involves profiling athletes to understand their performance testing and also identify their strengths and weaknesses.

These analyses include assessing the athlete's BMI, date of birth, gender, chronological age, biological age (i.e., maturity offset or the age of peak height velocity), technical training age, an athlete's strengths and weaknesses, and an athlete's injury history.

The athlete's objectives must also be assessed. What are their personal goals? What are the coach's goals for the athlete and the player-coach agreed goals?

3. Comparative analysis

After getting information on the sports and the athlete, the next thing is to compare both and identify how the athlete compares to the other athletes in that sport.

Challenges of a NEEDs analysis

The two main issues with NEEDs analysis in sports are lack of research data on a particular sport and overwhelming amounts of information, which may lead to over-complication.

How to conduct a NEEDs analysis

- Collect data on the athlete's current abilities, skill level, and performance.

- Identify areas for improvement.

- Design a training program that addresses the identified areas for improvement.

- Implement the program and monitor the athlete's progress.

- Assess the effectiveness of the training program.

Training Methods and Modes

There are several training methods used in exercise. They include:

- Bodyweight training method

- Core stability and balance training methods

- Variable-resistance training methods

- Nontraditional implement training methods

1. Bodyweight training method

This type of exercise uses your body weight as resistance. No equipment is used.

Some common methods of body weight training include:

A. Calisthenics: Calisthenics is a form of strength training that utilize body weight to perform movements. The exercises improve coordination, endurance, and mobility while strengthening muscles. Common examples include squats, push-ups, lunges, and crunches.

B. High-intensity interval training (HIIT): These types of workouts can be done using only bodyweight exercises, making them convenient for those who don't have access to gym equipment or who prefer to work out at home. HIIT consists of alternating between high-intensity exercises and periods of rest or lighter activity. Some HIIT exercises include running in place, mountain climbers, Burpees, high kicks, and more.

C. Progressive overload: Progressive overload involves gradually increasing the difficulty of a strength training routine to continue promoting muscle growth and avoiding adaptation. This can be achieved by increasing weight, reps, frequency, intensity, or endurance. Progressive overload helps to prevent plateaus and maintain progress in strength and fitness.

D. Circuit training: This form of exercise involves doing a sequence of exercises back-to-back without rest, repeated multiple times. It typically involves 5-to-10 different exercises, or stations, that target different muscle groups. The goal is to maintain a high heart rate by minimizing rest between exercises. Circuit training aims to provide a full-body workout in a short amount of time. A normal circuit will have five to ten different movements per circuit. This is often referred to as stations.

E. Unilateral training: Unilateral exercises are single-leg or single-arm movements that promote equal use of both sides of the body. This exercise helps to correct muscle imbalances, improve balance, engage core muscles, prevent injury, and aid in rehabilitation. Common examples of unilateral exercises include split squats, Romanian deadlifts, split lunges, single-arm pressing and rowing, single-leg, and pistol squats.

F. Isometric training: This method of training involves holding the muscle in a static position to build strength. Some examples of isometric exercises include wall sit, high plank hold, low squat, glute bridge, and side plank.

G. Split training: Split training involves dividing the body into different muscle groups and training each group on different days. This allows for greater focus on specific muscle groups and may also help to prevent overtraining.

<u>Benefits of Bodyweight Training</u>

- They are convenient

- They do not require any equipment; hence, they are cost-effective

- They improve functional fitness

- They improve flexibility and balance

- They are generally low-impact, and a good option for people with joint pain or injuries

- They are scalable

Limitations of bodyweight training

- They might not be enough resistance to challenge your muscles to get stronger

- It may be difficult to isolate some specific muscle groups

- Progression may be limited

- It may be difficult to achieve maximum strength gains

- It may become repetitive and boring over time

2. Core stability and balance training methods

The core refers to the center of the body and includes muscles that stabilize the hips, torso, and shoulders to provide stability during movement.

The term "core" is often used to refer to the trunk area of the body. The anatomical core typically includes the axial skeleton (including the pelvic and shoulder girdles) and the soft tissues that originate on it, such as muscles, tendons, ligaments, fascia, and articular cartilage.

These muscles play a role in generating force and resisting motion, and they allow for the transfer of torque and angular momentum during physical activities like kicking and throwing.

When an athlete's core stability is increased, it will result in a better foundation for force production in the upper and lower extremities, building strength within.

Core exercises engage one or more major muscle groups such as the chest, shoulders, back, hips, or thighs, and involve movement at two or more joints (multi-joint exercises). These exercises are given priority in exercise selection due to their direct impact on sports performance.

Common exercises for training the core include:

• Isolation exercises: This involves actions that isolate specific core muscles without the involvement of the limbs. These actions can be dynamic or isometric. Some examples of isolation exercises that work on the core include planks (prone and side planks) and bridges.

• Ground-based free-weight exercise: These exercises seem to activate the core muscles more strongly compared to conventional isolation exercises that target the core. In addition, these exercises can create an unstable environment to boost muscle endurance, coordination, and control, reducing the risk of lower back injuries. Examples of ground-based free exercise include Olympic lifts, squats, and deadlifts.

Other examples of exercises that work on improving core stability and balance include yoga and Pilates, unilateral exercise (such as single-leg deadlifts, step-ups, and pistol squats) and Tai Chi and Qigong.

• Assistant Exercises: Unlike the core exercises that target large muscle areas, assistance exercises generally target smaller muscle groups such as the upper arm, abs, calf, neck, forearm, lower back, or front lower leg and typically only involve one joint. They are viewed as less critical for enhancing athletic performance. When categorizing resistance training exercises as core or assistance, the shoulder joint (consisting of the glenohumeral and shoulder girdle) is considered one primary joint. The same goes for the spine, as in exercises such as abdominal crunches and back extensions.

3. Variable-resistance training methods

In athletic training, resistance can be in the form of constant or variable resistance. Constant resistance is where the resistance applied to the target muscle or muscle group does not change through the range of motion. On the other hand, variable resistance involves applying differing degrees of force to maintain constant resistance, challenging the muscle to work harder.

Variable resistance training involves using heavy chains and elastic bands to improve strength and power.

Variable resistance exercises are designed to maximize muscle activation and improve strength and power. This can be achieved through the use of equipment or techniques that change resistance during an exercise, such as bands or chains, adjusting weight on a machine, or altering leverage. Common exercises that use variable resistance include bench presses, squats, and deadlifts.

Variable resistance is typically performed using specialized machines that allow control of the entire movement. These machines can be designed for any muscle group in the body and have features such as cables, pulleys, or other devices to create variability, and the user is placed in a fixed position to prevent the recruitment of other muscle groups.

4. Nontraditional implement training methods

Nontraditional implement training uses unconventional equipment to challenge the body and enhance functional strength and conditioning. These methods include using sandbags, kettlebells, tires, medicine balls, Indian clubs, or everyday objects like bags of groceries or heavy backpacks.

The goal of this training is to increase functional strength and conditioning of the body.

Types of nontraditional implement training include:

A. The strong man training: This includes exercises like tire flipping, log lifting and farmers' walk.

- Tire flipping

Tire flipping is a strength and conditioning exercise that uses heavy-duty tires, such as truck tires, which can have additional weight added to match the athlete's strength levels.

The appropriate tire size is chosen based on the athlete's height, width, weight, and tire tread. In general, the tire should not be taller than the athlete's standing height, and the tread should be free from cuts, debris, and exposed metal.

In addition, tire width can impact an athlete's capacity to execute the flip. Narrow tires are harder for taller athletes, and wider tires are harder for shorter athletes.

There are three main techniques for tire flipping: The sumo, backlift style, and shoulders-against-the-tire technique.

The sumo style is performed with a wide sumo deadlift stance.

The backlift style is performed with a narrower stance, similar to a deadlift.

The shoulders-against-the-tire technique involves squatting behind the tire, placing the shoulders on it, and using a supinated grip to raise the tire. The movement is initiated by extending the knees and hips and plantar flexing the ankles to push the tire forward and up. The athlete moves forward by taking two or three steps and flips the tire over by striking it with the quadriceps and extending the arms.

However, the surface should be suitable for tire flipping, and the technique should include placing the chin and anterior deltoid on the tire and using a supinated grip with the arms extended but not locked out.

- The log lift

This is a popular exercise in strongman training. It is similar to the "clean" that involves lifting and moving a log with added weight.

Logs can be used to perform a variety of exercises such as the clean, press, jerk, row, squat, deadlift, and lunge.

Weight is usually added to the log using traditional plates, making it easier to add different weights. However, it's challenging to determine how much weight to use as there is limited research on the matter available.

Another variation of log lifting uses water as resistance, with the claim that the fluid movement inside will result in increased activation of stabilizer muscles, but there is no scientific evidence to support this.

- The farmers walk

This is another popular strongman exercise. Here, the athlete holds a load in each hand and walks forward.

It is considered a useful exercise as it involves unstable and awkward resistance that requires both unilateral and bilateral movements.

The farmer's walk can be performed using either static loads (e.g., heavy dumbbells) or variable loads (e.g., water-filled objects).

B. The kettle training

Kettlebells are best used as a general preparation exercise. This training is effective for developing maximal strength and jumping performance capacity.

There are two main types of kettlebells: cast iron and sports kettlebells.

Selecting the Right Exercises

Selecting exercises for a resistance training program involves making informed decisions by the strength and conditioning professional based on factors such as the different types of resistance training exercises, the physical demands of the sport, the athlete's exercise technique proficiency, available equipment, and available training time.

The following is a general guideline for selecting exercises:

- Start with the basics such as squats, lunges, and push-ups

- Include compound exercises like squats, deadlifts, presses, and rows. Consider your goals for the athlete

- Consider the athlete's strengths and weaknesses

Principles of Exercise Order

The order of exercises is determined by the principles of fatigue and priority, which are closely related.

Fatigability refers to how susceptible each exercise is to neuromuscular fatigue. For example, high-intensity exercises like plyometrics, ballistic, and maximum strength are more susceptible due to their demand on nervous system output and high physiological and psychological readiness.

The type of muscle fibers used in the exercise also affects fatigability, with fast-twitch muscle fibers being more prone to fatigue due to their high contractile force and speed. However, these fibers can only sustain high velocity and force for a short period of time.

Therefore, high-intensity exercises should be performed first in a training session. On the other hand, low-intensity, single-joint accessory exercises targeting smaller muscle groups can be performed later in the session as they are less likely to be affected by fatigue.

The second principle of exercise order is the principle of priority, and it is closely related to fatigability. This principle states that an athlete should perform their most important exercises when they have the most energy and resources to do so, usually at the beginning of a training session and after a proper warm-up.

If the primary goal is to develop maximum strength, heavy compound lifts should come before high-velocity training, even though this doesn't follow the principle of fatigability. This decision is made to prioritize the primary goal of maximum strength development.

In summary:

- Start with exercises that target large muscle groups such as legs, chest, and back.

- It is best to start with multi-joint exercises (squats and deadlifts) before single-joint exercises (bicep curls and leg extensions). This is because multi-joint exercises are more demanding and require more energy.

- Prioritize compound exercises over isolation exercises, as compound exercises are more demanding and will tire you out faster.

- Identify your main goal (whether it is to build strength or endurance) and prioritize it.

- Prioritize exercises that target the rehabilitation of the injured muscle, joint, tendons, and ligaments.

- Vary the order of exercises or add new exercises to your routine.

- Allow yourself enough rest and recovery time between sets and exercises.

Exercise Intensities

Exercise intensity refers to the amount of energy expended during physical activity. This can be measured using heart rate, rating of perceived exertion (RPE), or power output.

There are three main ways to classify exercise intensity:

A. Low intensity: Low-intensity exercise involves slow movements that result in a constant heart rate and no noticeable alteration in breathing. This type of exercise is often associated with activities like walking or stretching and is identified by a low heart rate and low rating of perceived exertion (RPE).

B. Moderate-intensity: Moderate-intensity exercise involves any exercise that elevates your heart rate, breathing rate, and body temperature, resulting in sweating. Activities like jogging or cycling fall under this category and are characterized by a noticeable increase in heart rate and a moderate RPE. The Centers for Disease Control and Prevention also included brisk walking at a speed of three miles per hour, water aerobics, and gardening as examples of moderate-intensity exercise.

C. High-intensity: High-intensity exercise is marked by a rapid increase in heart rate, breathing rate, and body temperature, leading to sweating. This type of exercise is seen in activities like sprinting or HIIT, and a person's heart rate and RPE increase significantly. Examples of vigorous-intensity activities, according to the CDC, include running, calisthenics, swimming, and jumping rope. The level of intensity may vary from person to person, depending on fitness level and experience.

<u>Training Volumes</u>

Training volume is the measure of the total amount of physical work performed during a workout session or over the course of an exercise program. It encompasses several factors, including the intensity of the exercise, which is determined by the weight used, the number of repetitions, and sets.

In addition, volume also includes the tempo or speed of the exercises, with slower movements placing more tension on muscle tissue. For endurance or energy system training, volume is determined by factors such as the distance covered and the pace of movement. The traditional way of measuring training volume is by calculating "total volume," which is the result of the formula sets x reps x load.

Mathematically,

Training volume = Sets (S) x reps (R) x load (L)

For example, if you do 5 sets of 10 reps with 195 pounds on the barbell bench press, your training volume for that exercise is 9,750 pounds (5 x 10 x 195).

Calculating training load

To calculate the appropriate training load, we can use the formula:

Training load = One-rep max x % of one-rep max

Example: An athlete's estimated one-rep max for the squat is 250 pounds. What is the appropriate training load for the client if the program calls for 60% of their one-rep max?

Training load = 250 pounds x 0.60 = 150 pounds

Therefore, the appropriate training load for the client in this case would be 150 pounds.

Rest Periods, Recovery and Unloading, and Training

Rest

Rest periods in exercise refer to the breaks taken between sets or exercises to allow the body to recover and prepare for the next set or activity. The length of these rest periods varies and depends on the type of workout, its intensity, and the individual's goals.

Short rest periods: This takes about 30-60 seconds and is used for high-intensity power exercises like weightlifting, plyometrics, or sprints for more reps in less time and to improve cardio fitness.

Medium rest periods: This takes about 1-2 minutes and is used for moderate-intensity activities like circuit training and compound exercises for adequate muscle recovery and endurance improvement.

Long rest periods: This takes about 2-5 minutes and is used for heavy low-rep exercises like powerlifting and strength training to prevent fatigue and injury.

Athletes who want to increase muscle size typically use short to moderate rest periods between sets of exercises.

Some training programs support shorter rest periods to continue the workout before full recovery is achieved.

However, the high intensity of exercises for large muscle groups might require more recovery time.

Common rest period lengths are less than 1.5 minutes or 30 seconds to 1 minute, or 30 seconds to 1.5 minutes.

On the other hand, muscular endurance training programs often have very short rest periods of less than 30 seconds, as light loads are lifted for multiple repetitions and minimal recovery time is allowed. This type of program is designed to meet the principle of specificity for muscular endurance and is common in circuit training programs.

Rest periods can be adjusted based on specific needs and goals, but it's important to allow adequate rest between workout sessions to avoid injury or burnout. A common guideline is to wait at least 48 hours before training the same muscle group again.

Recovery

Exercise recovery involves giving the body time to heal and adjust to the demands of physical exertion.

There are three methods of recovery: the primary, secondary, and tertiary methods. The primary method of recovery includes eating a well-balanced diet, proper hydration, and getting enough sleep.

The secondary method of recovery includes dynamic stretching, low-intensity cardio exercise, low-intensity full range of motion lifts, and soft tissue modalities like myofascial release.

The tertiary methods of recovery include cryotherapy, compression, and massage.

Unloading

Unloading involves temporarily lowering the level of intensity, volume, or frequency of a workout to promote recovery and prevent overtraining.

Unloading can enhance overall fitness by preventing muscle and joint overuse, promoting recovery, overcoming plateaus in fitness, and correcting muscle imbalances caused by overtraining.

Unloading should not be mistaken for detraining, which is a complete stop to exercise. Unloading can be achieved by reducing weight, reps, sets, frequency of workout, or taking a break from a specific exercise.

The duration of the unloading phase in a periodized training program can vary based on factors such as the athlete's training history, goals, and current level of fatigue.

Overreaching

Overreaching is a short-term decrease in performance that typically resolves itself within a week or two. When properly planned, overreaching can be incorporated into a training regimen to achieve a "supercompensation" effect, which results in increased power and strength.

Detraining

Detraining refers to the decline in performance that occurs when training stops, or there is a significant decrease in the volume, intensity, or frequency of training.

It is important to note that detraining does not result in immediate performance loss, and there is a lag time before the decrease in performance becomes noticeable.

Exercise Progression

Exercise progression is the gradual increase in intensity, duration, or complexity of an exercise program with the aim of improving physical fitness and reaching specific goals. It is an important technique that helps athletes maintain an effective and well-rounded workout routine, allowing the body to adapt to new physical demands and improve muscle strength, endurance, and overall health.

There are several ways to achieve exercise progression. One can increase the weight in strength training, distance, or speed in cardio, add more complex movements, or increase the duration of the workout.

It is best to start with lower resistance or intensity levels and then gradually increase. Varying the types of workouts to balance the workload on different muscle groups is also important to prevent overuse injuries. By gradually increasing the intensity, duration, or complexity of an exercise, the body can adapt and continue to improve fitness levels, leading to improved overall health and well-being.

Periodization Models and Concepts

Periodization is a technique in exercise training that involves breaking down the training program into specific phases or periods, each with its own specific focus and goal. The goal of periodization is to optimize performance and reduce the risk of injury by systematically varying the training load and intensity over time.

Types of periodization models

There are several periodization models, including linear periodization, block periodization, undulating periodization, conjoint periodization, functional periodization, and reversed periodization.

Linear periodization: In this model, training volume and intensity are gradually increased over time with the goal of peaking for a specific event or competition.

Block periodization: This model entails dividing the training program into time blocks, each with a distinct focus and goal. For example, one block could focus on strength training while another on endurance training.

Conjoint periodization: This model entails combining various periodization models, such as linear and undulating periodization, to target specific fitness components and optimize performance.

Undulating periodization: In this model, training volume and intensity are alternated on a daily or weekly basis rather than gradually increasing over time. This can aid in the prevention of plateaus and the enhancement of overall fitness.

Functional periodization: This training model involves training the body to mimic the specific movements and demands of a sport or activity.

Reverse periodization: This model begins with a high-intensity and low-volume and gradually decreases the intensity while increasing the volume over time. It is more commonly used in power and strength sports.

The choice of model will depend on the individual's goals, schedule, and specific sport or activity. It is important to consult with a coach or sports performance professional to ensure that the periodization model chosen is appropriate and effective.

Periodization cycles

In addition, periodization can be divided into three main cycles: microcycle, mesocycle, and macrocycle.

The microcycle is the shortest cycle, typically lasting one to two weeks, and is used to organize daily and weekly training schedules.

The mesocycle is a medium-length cycle, typically lasting several weeks to a few months, and is used to focus on specific training goals and objectives.

The macrocycle is the longest cycle, typically lasting several months to a year, and is used to plan and organize the overall training program.

The cycles used in periodization are not mutually exclusive and may overlap, depending on the periodization model used.

For example, in linear periodization, the macrocycle is usually divided into mesocycles, each with a specific focus, such as endurance, strength, and power.

In block periodization, the macrocycle is divided into several blocks, each with a specific focus, such as strength, power, or endurance.

In undulating periodization, the macrocycle is divided into several mesocycles, each with a specific focus, such as endurance, strength, and power.

Incorporating sport seasons into the periodization cycles

Off-Season: This is considered the preparation period. It usually lasts from the end of the post-season to the start of the pre-season, which could be around six weeks prior to the first major competition (although this may vary significantly).

Pre-Season: This leads to the first competition and usually includes the final stages of the preparation period and the first transition period with a focus on the strength/power phase of resistance training.

In-Season: Comprises all the competitions scheduled for that year, including any tournament matches.

Post-Season: Follows the final competition.

Central concepts related to periodization

A. General Adaptation Syndrome (GAS): This concept describes the body's physiological response to stressors. It has three stages: alarm, resistance, and exhaustion.

In the alarm phase, a new stress is introduced. In addition, the body responds to the perceived threat with a "fight or flight" response, including an increase in adrenaline and other stress hormones. The resistance stage is characterized by the continuation of the stress response, with the body's stress hormones remaining elevated. This is the phase where an athlete will start to adapt to new stressors and may experience supercompensation. In the last phase, the exhaustion stage, the body's resources are depleted, resulting in physical and mental exhaustion.

B. Stimulus-fatigue-recovery-adaptation theory: This theory is an extension of the GAS theory. According to this theory, the intensity of the workout influences the response to training. The more difficult the workout, the more fatigue is built up and the longer it takes for full recovery and adaptation to occur. If no new training is introduced, the body will begin to detrain. The process is repeated when a new training stimulus is introduced.

C. Fitness-fatigue paradigm: The fitness-fatigue paradigm is a classic explanation of the relationships between fitness and fatigue following training interventions, as well as their impact on the athlete's level of preparedness.

Each training session or cycle produces both fitness and fatigue effects, which add up to produce a state of preparedness. When training loads are high, fitness improves, but fatigue rises, reducing readiness. Low training loads, on the other hand, result in little fatigue and fitness, resulting in a lack of preparedness. The sequencing of training loads is critical for varying training loads in a systematic manner.

Fatigue disappears at a faster rate than fitness. Because fatigue fades faster than fitness, training strategies that maintain fitness while reducing fatigue can improve preparedness. Depending on the structure of the periodized training plan, the residual training effects of one training period can impact the level of preparedness in subsequent training periods.

D. Supercompensation: This refers to the period after training when an athlete's performance has surpassed their previous level before the training period. Supercompensation is a process by which the body adapts to the stress of exercise by overcompensating for the stress and becoming stronger and more resistant to future stress. The process of supercompensation involves a temporary increase in the body's physiological and biochemical adaptations, including an increase in muscle glycogen storage, muscle protein synthesis, and overall muscle fiber size and strength.

Injury/Reconditioning Period

The injury and reconditioning phase of physical activity entails recovering from an injury or illness and working toward regaining physical fitness, strength, and flexibility.

It is important to collaborate with a medical professional or physical therapist to develop a customized exercise plan that promotes healing and prevents future injuries.

The goal of this phase is to gradually progress exercises to regain muscle strength, range of motion, and overall fitness, which may include flexibility, balance, core stability, and muscle strengthening exercises. To avoid reinjury, resistance or intensity levels should begin slowly and gradually increase with proper form and technique.

Physical therapy, massage therapy, chiropractic care, and acupuncture may be used during the injury and reconditioning phase to help relieve pain and improve mobility.

Organization and Administration

Organizational Environment

The strength and conditioning profession requires a combination of sports knowledge, exercise science knowledge, administration, management, teaching, and coaching skills. The strength and conditional specialists must also follow laws and regulations and handle injury incidents and related legal issues. This makes it a challenging field that requires expertise, experience, and resources, especially in multi-sport environments like colleges and schools.

Strength and conditioning specialists work with athletes of varying abilities and also with non-athletes looking to enhance their physical attributes such as strength, speed, agility, and stamina.

Strength and conditioning coaches can work either inside, like in a gym or fitness center, or outside, like by a swimming pool. Those working with college or professional sports teams may have a demanding schedule, working up to 60 hours a week, including evenings and weekends during the competition season. Some travel may be necessary for games away from home.

The staff-to-athlete ratio in junior high strength and conditioning facilities should not exceed 1:10. In addition, the ratio of high school facilities to students should not exceed 1:15, and a 1:20 ratio should be maintained in college.

A strength and conditioning specialist (SCS) should be familiar with the organization in which they work. Here are a few key areas in which a SCS should be knowledgeable:

• The organization's mission and goals: Understanding the organization's mission and goals can assist a SCS in aligning the strength and conditioning program with the organization's overall objectives.

• The organization's culture and values: Understanding the organization's culture and values can assist a SCS in developing a program that is consistent with the organization's beliefs and values and will be embraced by the athletes and staff.

• The budget and resources: Understanding the strength and conditioning program's resources and budget can help a SCS make informed decisions about equipment and staffing, as well as prioritize spending.

• The organizational structure: Understanding the organization structure can assist a SCS in identifying key stakeholders, such as the head coach, athletic director, and other decision-makers, and communicating effectively with them.

- Organizational policies and procedures: Understanding organizational policies and procedures can assist a SCS in ensuring that the strength and conditioning program adheres to all applicable laws, regulations, and guidelines.

- Organizational legal and liability issues: Understanding the organization legal and liability issues can assist a SCS in minimizing the risk of injury and liability for the organization.

- Organizational trends and best practices in strength and conditioning: Understanding organizational trends and best practices in strength and conditioning can assist a SCS in staying current and implementing best practices in their program.

Assessing athletic program needs

The needs and requirements of the athletes and sport are the most important aspects of facility design and layout.

Facility designers should be able to answer the following questions:

- How many athletes will use the facility?

- What are the training objectives for the athletes, coaches, and administration?

- What are the demographics of the athletes?

- How will the athletes' training experience be?

- How will the athletes be scheduled?

- What equipment needs to be repaired or modified?

Design, Layout, and Organization of the Strength and Conditioning Facility

Designing a new strength and conditioning facility involves four main phases, including:

- The pre-design phase
- The design phase
- Construction phase
- Pre-operation phase

A. The pre-design phase: This phase usually takes up 25% of the total project duration (6 months). The primary focus is conducting a needs analysis and feasibility study to determine costs, location, and programs of interest. It also entails assessing the facility's needs and goals, such as the type of athletes or clients who will use the facility, the types of training and equipment that will be required, and the overall budget and space constraints.

B. The design phase: This phase may consume 10-12% of the total project time (around three months), where the coach works with an architect to finalize plans, determine equipment needs, and design the facility for user-friendly access for all athletes.

C. The construction phase: This phase typically takes 50% of the total project time (12 months) and requires strict adherence to set deadlines. It involves creating detailed plans and specifications for the facility, including drawings, equipment lists, and detailed cost estimates.

D. The pre-operation phase: Also known as the start-up phase, the pre-operation phase requires about 15% of the total project duration (3-4 months) and focuses on staffing considerations. This phase also includes testing and commissioning the facility, as well as training staff and athletes on how to use the equipment properly.

Existing strength and conditioning facilities

Modifying an existing strength and conditioning facility is similar to designing a new one, but without the process of building from scratch. In some cases, the modification process can be lengthy.

A committee can also be formed for an existing facility; however, members such as a contractor and an architect may not be necessary. The hiring process for an existing facility may also differ. Sometimes, strength and conditioning professionals continue to work in the same facility even after changes in ownership or management. Nonetheless, there should still be a focus on standards, education, professionalism, and staff development. The strength and conditioning professional should evaluate the existing equipment based on the needs of all athletes and teams who use the facility.

Designing a strength and conditioning facility

When setting up a strength and conditioning facility, consider key design factors such as location, access, structure, environment, and safety to ensure optimal functionality and user experience.

Here are some considerations to keep in mind when designing a strength and conditioning facility:

Location: The ideal location for a strength and conditioning facility is on the ground floor, away from offices and classrooms to minimize noise disruptions. The floor must be able to support heavy equipment with a load-bearing capacity of at least 100 lbs per sq. ft. if not located on the ground floor.

Supervision location: For optimal supervision, the facility manager's office should be centrally located and equipped with clear views and mirrors to monitor activity throughout the weight room. An elevated office position provides an improved vantage point.

Accessibility: The facility must be accessible for people with disabilities, with a ramp or wheelchair lift for any changes in height exceeding 0.5 inches (13 mm). The ramp should have a 12-inch run for every 1-inch rise, and steps should have a rough strip to prevent falls.

A mechanical lift or elevator can also be used for accessibility. The weight room should have double doors for easy movement of equipment, but if the hallway is too narrow, the size of the doors will not matter, and an outside wall may need to be temporarily removed or a garage door opened for equipment transfer.

Ceiling height: The ceiling height should allow for jumping and explosive activities, including the athlete's height, and additional space for exercises such as box jumps, vertical jumps, and Olympic lifting. A recommended ceiling height is 12-14 feet, providing enough clearance for athletes to perform these activities comfortably

Flooring: Strength and conditioning facilities have various flooring options, including rubber flooring and antifungal carpet, or indoor turf for plyometric, agility, and conditioning exercises for ground-based movements and sled pushes.

Rubber flooring, though more expensive, is easier to clean and comes in rolls, insert tiles, or a poured surface. Ideal weightlifting platforms have a wooden center for safe lifting and rubber outer sections to prevent shoes from getting caught or sliding.

Environmental factors: The lighting in the facility should consist of both artificial and natural light, with a brightness of 50-100 lumens, depending on ceiling height and natural light. Natural light sources, such as windows and mirrors, can improve the facility's appearance. The temperature should be kept between 68°F to 78°F (20-25 °C) and relative humidity not exceeding 60% to prevent bacteria growth. The HVAC system should have the ability to control temperature in different areas of the facility, and air exchange should occur 8-to-12 times per hour for comfort and to prevent stagnant air. Circulation can be achieved through HVAC, fresh air exchange, and fans (2-4 per 1,200 sq. ft).

Sound systems: A sound system can enhance the training environment by providing motivation through music. However, the volume should be less than 90 decibels. In addition, speakers should be elevated and placed in a corner, and background noise should be reduced through sound-absorbing material in the floors and walls, especially for yoga or dance classes.

Electrical Service: A strength and conditioning facility needs more electrical outlets compared to other buildings. Some outlets may need a higher voltage to accommodate powerful equipment such as stair climbers, elliptical machines, and treadmills. The electrical service must be grounded properly to prevent damage from lightning strikes or power surges. Ground-fault circuits are necessary to ensure safety in case of an electrical short.

Mirrors: Mirrors in a strength and conditioning facility can serve dual purposes. They can be used as a coaching tool by providing immediate visual feedback to athletes and also improve the room's aesthetic by reflecting light. Mirrors should be positioned at least 6 inches away from equipment and 20 inches above the floor to avoid damage from dropped weights or plates.

Other considerations for a strength and conditioning facility include a drinking fountain located away from the training area, locker rooms with showers for hygiene, a phone accessible to those in wheelchairs for safety, bumper rails or padding for protection of surfaces, and a storage room for equipment and supplies. The size of the storage room depends on the size of the facility and the amount of equipment.

<u>Arranging equipment in the strength and conditioning facility</u>

The arrangement of equipment in a strength and conditioning facility is crucial for safety and efficiency. Equipment should be grouped into sections, including a stretching and warm-up area, agility and plyometrics, free weights, aerobic area, and resistance machines.

Free weights and racks: Free weights and racks should be organized along a wall, with walkways between them to prevent congestion and maximize space.

Machines: Machines can be lined up in the middle of the room, with tall machines bolted to the floor or a wall. Cardiorespiratory machines should be in their own section, grouped together and away from the walkways.

Barbells and dumbbells: Barbells and dumbbells need at least 36 inches of space between them, with weight trees placed close to plate-loaded equipment.

Racks: Racks are best placed along a wall with at least 36 inches of space around them. Smaller equipment is better placed in the middle of the room for visibility, and bigger equipment can be bolted to the walls. Traffic flow is influenced by equipment placement, with walkways created by arranging equipment in a row running the length of the facility.

Stretching and warm-up area: The stretching and warm-up area should have soft tissue instruments, mats, or bands, and at least 49 square feet of open space.

Circuit training area: The machines in a circuit training setup should have a minimum separation of 24 inches (61 cm) and optimally 36 inches (91 cm) for a spacious walking area and a safety buffer. The walkways within the circuit training area should measure between four-to-seven feet (1.2-2.1 m) for comfortable movement.

Free weights: Free weights equipment, including dumbbells, barbells, and squat racks, should be lined up along a wall, with enough room for movement and safety.

Weightlifting area: A weightlifting area typically includes racks with platforms or just a standalone platform. In some cases, it may be an open space for weightlifting without a platform, usually on a rubber floor over a concrete base. Racks and platforms should be spaced three-to-four feet (0.9-1.2 m) apart to avoid injury in case of a fall. The weightlifting racks should also be securely bolted to the floor to prevent movement during use. Portable racks should be stored in a designated area when not in use.

Aerobic area: The aerobic area houses cardiopulmonary training equipment such as stationary bikes, stair climbers, ellipticals, treadmills, and rowers. 24 ft2 is required for bikes and stair machines, 45 ft2 for treadmills, and 40 ft2 for rowers.

These measurements include the necessary space between machines.

Maintaining and cleaning surfaces and equipment

Strength and conditioning facilities should be regularly cleaned and maintained to ensure safe training and protect investments. Surfaces should be wiped down with germicidal cleaners and equipment should be checked for broken or damaged parts.

A cleaning schedule should be made for daily, weekly, bi-weekly, or monthly cleaning of equipment. Furthermore, cleaning and maintenance materials should be kept in storage, locked, and inventoried regularly. Tools should be kept in a toolbox and out of sight.

Professional Practice

The scope of practice of a strength and conditioning professional refers to the range of activities and responsibilities that a qualified professional is authorized to perform within their specific field.

A strength and conditioning professional is typically in charge of designing and implementing safe and effective strength and conditioning programs for athletes and clients of all ages and skill levels. This includes:

Conducting assessments: This involves assessing an individual's physical capabilities, such as flexibility, strength, power, speed, and endurance, and using this information to design a personalized training program.

Supervising exercises: Strength and conditioning specialists are also responsible for demonstrating exercises and techniques. They also monitor form, and provide feedback and correction as needed to ensure that exercises are performed safely and effectively.

Monitoring progress: The strength and conditioning specialist also monitors an individual's progress over time, making necessary changes to the training program, and providing feedback and encouragement to help the individual achieve their goals.

Creating training programs: The strength and conditioning profession is responsible for designing and implementing safe and effective strength and conditioning programs that are tailored to the specific needs of the athletes or clients.

Educating and advising: This includes educating and advising athletes, clients, and other professionals on topics like proper exercise technique, injury prevention, and nutrition.

Professional development: The strength and conditioning professional must dedicate themselves to continued education. They should also participate in professional development courses and keep abreast of the most recent research in the field.

Strength and conditioning professionals should become acquainted with the NSCA Code of Ethics as well as their institution's code of ethics, and if applicable, the student-athlete code of conduct.

<u>Emergency Response Plan</u>

Key components of the emergency response plan include:

- Emergency medical services activation process

- Contact information for primary, secondary, and tertiary emergency contacts

- Exact location of the strength and conditioning center for emergency responders

- Telephone location

- Nearest exits

- Designated personnel trained to provide medical care

- Access to ambulance

- Location of emergency supplies and first aid kit

- Action plan for various emergencies, such as fires, tornadoes, life-threatening injuries, crimes, and acts of terrorism

Keep in mind that in the event of a fire in a strength and conditioning facility, the first step that should be taken is to evacuate the building immediately. The safety of all individuals in the facility is the top priority, and everyone should be instructed to leave the building as quickly and safely as possible.

Disciplinary Committee

The discipline system in place involves a tiered penalty system. For the first offense, the staff member will give a verbal warning. If a second offense occurs, the person will be dismissed from the facility for a day, and the offense will be documented. If there is a third offense, the person will be dismissed for a week. For a fourth offense, the person will be dismissed for the rest of the year, and for the fifth offense, they will be permanently dismissed from the facility.

Legal Issues

Strength and conditioning professionals have legal duties to provide safe and appropriate training programs, ensure equipment safety and maintenance, stay current with the latest research, and provide appropriate progressions for athletes with injuries or conditions.

They must also inform participants of inherent risks and prevent unreasonable harm from negligent instruction or supervision. Participants assume the risk of injury through voluntary participation with knowledge of the risks.

If a strength and conditioning professional fails to meet these duties and causes injury, they may be held liable for negligence. The standard of care is to act as a reasonable and prudent person with their education, training, and certification. They have a responsibility to manage risk and should involve all facility staff in the process.

Strength and conditioning experts must familiarize themselves with prohibited drugs and substances as athletes often seek their guidance, and the misuse of such substances can lead to disqualification from competitions.

In addition, strength and conditioning professionals must not prescribe, recommend, or provide illegal, prohibited, or harmful drugs, controlled substances, or supplements to participants for any purpose, including enhancing athletic performance, physique, or conditioning.

Risk management

Risk management is a proactive process that aims to reduce legal liability, cut down on the number and severity of injuries and claims, and keep a company from being sued.

The 4-step procedure for applying standards of practice to risk management in strength and conditioning involves:

- Identifying and selecting relevant standards

- Developing risk management strategies

- Implementing the plan

- Evaluating the plan regularly

The NSCA has identified nine areas of liability exposure in strength and conditioning and eleven standards and fourteen guidelines have been established to guide practitioners in reducing risk.

Legal terms to be familiar with in strength and conditioning:

Risk Management: Strategies to reduce legal liability through controlling the risk of injury.

Informed consent: A process where risks are explained to participants and they make an informed decision to participate.

Liability: Legal responsibility, obligation, or duty.

Negligence: Failure to act as a reasonable person, includes duty, breach of duty, proximate cause, and damages.

Standard of care: What a reasonable person would do in similar circumstances.

Duty: Responsibility to act.

Breach of duty: Failure to fulfill the responsibility to act with appropriate care.

Proximate cause: An event linked to an injury that a court determines to be responsible for.

Damages: Physical or economic harm.

Assumption of risk: Acknowledgement of inherent risk in participating and choosing to participate anyway.

Scope of practice: Procedures, actions, and processes authorized by professional licensing.

Facility usage: Criteria established for training population and prearranged schedules for other groups/individuals.

Statute of limitations: The time frame to file a lawsuit—varies by state and country. Highlights the importance of record keeping.

Liability insurance: Recommended for strength and conditioning professionals due to the risk of injury.

Product liability: Legal responsibility of manufacturer/seller if harm occurs from product use. Professionals may be held liable if a product is changed or used inappropriately.

Disciplinary paperwork: Athletes may need to sign documentation acknowledging they will follow facility rules/guidelines.

Testing, ongoing monitoring, and data evaluation

Key terms you should know:

Test: A method for determining proficiency in a specific task.

Field test: A test performed outside the laboratory environment, which does not require specialized training or costly equipment.

Measurement: The process of gathering information through a test.

Evaluation: The evaluation of test results to make informed decisions.

Pre-test: A test taken before the start of training to determine the individual's baseline abilities.

Mid-Test: A test administered during the training period to monitor progress and make adjustments to the program for optimal results.

Formative evaluation: Regular reevaluations based on progress tests conducted during the training.

Post-test: A test taken after the completion of training to determine the effectiveness of the training program in achieving its goals.

<u>Evidence-Based Tests to Maximize Test Reliability and Validity</u>

<u>Test for reliability</u>

Reliability refers to consistency of test results and can be ensured by using standardized administration procedures, clear instructions, and a suitable test.

There are several types of reliability tests that can be used to assess results consistency, including:

Retest reliability: This type of reliability test involves administering the same test to the same group of people twice and comparing the results. This test is used to assess the consistency of test results over time.

Alternate-form reliability: This involves administering two different versions of the same test to the same group of people and then comparing the results. This type of reliability test is used to assess the consistency of test scores when different versions of the test are administered.

Split-half reliability: This type of reliability test involves giving half of the test items to one group of people and the other half to another group of people, and then comparing the results. When different subsets of the test are used, this type of reliability is used to measure the consistency of scores.

Inter-rater reliability: In this type of testing, multiple raters will score the same test results and then compare the results to see how consistent they are. This type of reliability test is especially useful when assessing the consistency of scores when the test is scored by different raters.

Intra-class correlation: This test compares the similarity of scores from different raters or different test forms. This type of reliability test assesses the consistency of scores across raters or test forms.

Alpha of Cronbach: This type of reliability test is a statistical method for determining test score internal consistency. This type of reliability test is also used to assess the consistency of test scores.

Test for validity

Validity refers to the extent to which the test measures what it's intended to measure and can be ensured by using multiple measures (self-report, observational, objective), and ensuring the test is specific to the sport and measures important variables.

Types of validity include:

1. Criterion-referenced validity: Criterion-related validity is used to determine the relationship between a test and a criterion measure, such as performance in a sport-specific task or competition. There are three types of criterion-referenced validity: Concurrent, predictive, and discriminant.

a. Concurrent validity: Concurrent validity is used to determine the relationship between a test and another measure that is currently in use.

b. Predictive validity: Predictive validity is used to determine the ability of a test to predict future performance in a sport. The effectiveness of a test score in predicting success in a sport can be determined by comparing the test score with actual performance in the sport.

c. Discriminant validity: Discriminant validity is a property of a test that allows it to differentiate between two distinct constructs. This is shown by the low correlation between the test's results and the results of tests measuring a different construct.

2. Face validity: Face validity refers to the perceived accuracy of a test or test item by the athlete and other casual observers. When a test has face validity, the athlete is more likely to have a positive attitude toward it. The evaluation of face validity is typically informal and non-quantitative.

3. Construct validity: Construct validity is used to determine the relationship between a test and other constructs or variables related to the sport. Construct validity is a term used to describe the overall accuracy of a test. It also refers to the degree to which the test accurately measures the concept or ability it was intended to assess.

4. Content validity: Content validity is used to ensure that a test covers the entire range of the construct or variable being measured.

5. Convergent validity: Convergent validity refers to the degree to which a test used by strength and conditioning professionals matches the results of a widely accepted standard. A test may be considered a gold standard if it demonstrates convergent validity with the standard while being more efficient in terms of time, equipment, cost, or technical knowledge required.

Order of tests

- Non-fatiguing tests
- Tests of agility
- Tests of maximum power and strength
- Tests of sprinting ability
- Tests of local muscular endurance
- Tests of fatiguing anaerobic capacity
- Tests of aerobic endurance

Statistical Analysis of Test Results

Descriptive statistics

- Central measures
- Mean: the average of all scores
- Median: the middle score when scores are ordered by magnitude
- Mode: the score that appears most frequently

Variability

- Range: the difference between the highest and lowest score

- Standard deviation: a measure of how much scores deviate from the mean

- Percentile rank: the percentage of test takers with a lower score than an individual

Inferential statistics: This is used to make general conclusions about a population from a sample. The Sample must be representative of the population.

Magnitude statistics: This can provide a useful interpretation of fitness test results. Here, the smallest significant change is the smallest meaningful improvement in performance that can be detected by a test

Effect Size (ES): This is a statistic that helps to compare the performance change between groups of athletes or after a training program.

ES = (post-test score - pre-test score) / pre-test standard deviation

Monitoring Protocols and Procedures

Monitoring protocols and procedures in sports are methods and techniques used to track and measure an athlete's performance, health, and well-being over time.

This process entails taking repeated measurements of an athlete in order to provide relevant data to guide the training process.

Some important testing that you should know include:

- Anthropometrics: Measures height, weight, body mass index (BMI), waist circumference, and body fat percentage.

- Physiological: Measures heart rate, blood pressure, respiratory rate, oxygen uptake, and lactate threshold.

- Mechanical stress: Measures joint loading, impact forces, and shear forces.

- Muscular strength: Typically measured through 1-repetition maximum (1RM) tests.

- Muscular power: Measured through vertical jump tests or other power-based movements.

- Aerobic capacity: Typically measured through maximal oxygen uptake (VO2max) tests.

- Anaerobic capacity: Typically measured through tests such as the Wingate Anaerobic Test.

- Muscular endurance: Typically measured through tests such as maximum push-up or sit-up tests.

- Agility: Typically measured through tests such as the T-Test or the Pro Agility Test.

Evaluating and Interpreting Results

The process of analyzing and making sense of data collected from monitoring protocols and procedures is referred to as evaluating and interpreting results in sports. This procedure consists of several steps, including:

Data collection: This is the process of collecting information from monitoring protocols and procedures such as physical measurements, performance tests, and injury and wellness assessments.

Data processing: This involves organizing and cleaning the data, such as removing outliers, calculating averages, and creating charts and graphs.

Data analysis: This process involves identifying patterns and trends in data using statistical methods, such as identifying changes in performance over time or identifying risk factors for injury.

Data interpretation: This refers to the process of making sense of data, such as determining the implications of the data for the athlete's training and recovery, as well as making recommendations for future actions.

Communicating the results: This final step entails sharing the results with the appropriate stakeholders, such as coaches, trainers, and medical professionals, as well as discussing the implications of the results for the athlete's training and performance.

Test 1 Questions

1. Which of the following organs is responsible for the generation of sounds for speech?

A. Pharynx

B. Larynx

C. Trachea

D. Epiglottis

2. Which of the following components of the muscle detects changes in the length of a muscle?

A. Axon

B. Dendrites

C. Muscle spindles

D. Synaptic cleft

3. What is the term used to describe the process through which blood cells are produced in the bone marrow?

A. Hematopoiesis

B. Leukopoiesis

C. Erythropoiesis

D. Thrombopoiesis

4. In a setting similar to a college or university, what is the recommended ratio of coaches to athletes when the weight room is in high demand?

A. 1:7

B. 1:13

C. 1:20

D. 1:21

5. Which of the following substances acts at the neuromuscular junction to excite the muscle fibers of a motor unit?

A. Troponin

B. Acetylcholine

C. Acetylcholinesterase

D. Creatine phosphate

6. The left and right lungs are separated by a compartment called _____.

A. Diaphragm

B. Pleural cavity

C. Mediastinum

D. Pleural membrane

7. The following are physiologic functions that occur with aging, except _____.

A. Reduced cardiac output

B. Increased maximal heart rate

C. Reduced oxygen level

D. Reduced stroke volume

8. Which of the following sports is typically considered to be easier to excel in for teenage girls compared to teenage boys?

A. Football

B. Basketball

C. Gymnastics

D. Weightlifting

9. The human muscle will stop contracting when all of the following happen, except when _____.

A. Calcium is pumped back into the sarcoplasmic reticulum

B. Acetylcholine is released

C. ATP stores are depleted

D. Muscle cells are fatigued

10. For an athlete running a light marathon, which of the following is the most probable limiting factor?

A. Liver glycogen

B. Muscle glycogen

C. Fat stores

D. ATP

11. All of these statements are true about anabolic reactions, except _____.

A. They are usually exergonic reactions

B. This type of reaction breaks down energy-storing molecules

C. Respiration is an example of an anabolic reaction

D. They require energy from the system

12. Which of the following is true about the phosphagen energy system?

A. It is one of the slowest ways to resynthesize ATP

B. The phosphagen system is oxygen dependent

C. This system uses carbohydrates or fat to generate ATP.

D. This energy system is instantaneously available.

13. Nerve fibers that carry signals from the spinal cord to effector organs are referred to as _____.

A. Axons

B. Dendrites

C. Muscle spindles

D. Synaptic cleft

14. The normal heart beats of an adult is _____.

A. 100-150 beats/min

B. 60-80 beats/min

C. 40-60 beats/min

D. 50-200 beats/min

15. The mediastinum houses all of the following organs, except _____.

A. Heart

B. Lungs

C. Thymus

D. Esophagus

16. Which of the following is a key mechanism responsible for the increase in muscle size and strength during strength training?

A. Increasing aerobic metabolism

B. Promoting protein synthesis

C. Increasing muscle fiber activation

D. Increased store ATP

17. What is the primary function of Purkinje fibers in the human heart?

A. Secreting hormones

B. Filtering blood

C. Conducting electrical impulses

D. Absorbing nutrients

18. Which of the following is an example of an isometric exercise?

A. Plank

B. Bicep curl

C. Leg press

D. Push-up

19. Muscle fascicles are surrounded by _____.

A. Perimysium

B. Epimysium

C. Endomysium

D. Mesomysium

20. Which energy system is primarily responsible for providing energy during high-intensity, short-duration activities lasting around 10 seconds?

A. Oxidative

B. Glycolytic

C. Phosphagen

D. None of the above

21. What is the primary role of carbohydrates in an athlete's diet?

A. To provide energy for physical activity

B. To promote muscle growth and repair

C. To support hormone production and regulation

D. To serve as a primary source of dietary fiber

22. Which principle of biomechanics states that energy can be transferred across body segments and joints in a system of linked bodies?

A. The principle of Optimal Projection

B. The principle of Segmental Interaction

C. The principle of Coordination Continuum

D. The principle of Range of Motion

23. What is the ideal work-rest ratio for a system powered by the Fast Glycolytic energy system?

A. 1:3 to 1:5

B. 1:12 to 1:20

C. 1:20 to 1:30

D. 1:1 to 1:3

24. Which of the following theories suggests that arousal helps performance up to a certain point, but if arousal goes beyond that point, it can start to hurt performance?

A. Inverted-U theory

B. Catastrophe theory

C. Drive theory

D. Arousal regulation theory

25. Which of the following statements is true?

I. Type IIx fibers are more prone to fatigue than type I

II. Type IIx fibers have a rich supply of blood capillaries

III. Competitive swimmers usually have high amounts of type I fibers

IV. Type IIa fibers are capable of anaerobic respiration.

A. I, II and III

B. II and III

C. I only

D. I and IV

26. The Valsalva maneuver is characterized by which of the following actions?

A. Rapid inhalation and exhalation

B. Forceful exhalation against a closed glottis

C. Hyperventilation

D. Breathing deeply and slowly

27. Which of the following muscle types is NOT striated?

A. Skeletal muscle

B. Cardiac muscle

C. Smooth muscle

D. All of the above are striated

28. What is the plasma membrane of a muscle fiber called?

A. Sarcolemma

B. Sarcoplasmic reticulum

C. Perimysium

D. Endomysium

29. Which of the following is a muscle found in the neck?

A. Trapezius

B. Pectoralis major

C. Sternocleidomastoid

D. Rectus abdominis

30. Which type of exercise involves low-repetition movements against high resistance?

A. Isotonic exercise

B. Isometric exercise

C. Aerobic exercise

D. Endurance exercise

31. Which type of exercise targets aerobic metabolism and improves fatigue resistance?

A. Strength training

B. Endurance training

C. Flexibility training

D. Power training

32. What is the recommended percentage of an athlete's daily caloric intake that should come from dietary fat?

A. 10-15%

B. 20-35%

C. 45-65%

D. 5-10%

33. What is bone remodeling?

A. The process of replacing an old bone with a new bone

B. The process of breaking down bone and bone tissue

C. The process of maintaining skeletal structure

D. The process of development of new bone

34. What factor affects how the neuromuscular system adapts to exercise?

A. The type of exercise

B. The frequency of exercise

C. The intensity of exercise

D. All of the above

35. Which principle of biomechanics states that before motion can occur, some forces must act first?

A. The principle of inertia

B. The principle of range of motion

C. The principle of balance

D. The principle of force-motion

36. During a barbell squat, which of the following are agonist muscles?

A. Transverse abdominus

B. Internal oblique

C. Quadriceps

D. Rectus abdominis

37. In which part of the cell does fatty acid oxidation occur?

A. Mitochondria

B. Ribosome

C. Cytoplasm

D. Nucleus

38. The thick structural protein found inside the sarcomere is called:

A. Actin

B. Sarcoplasm

C. Sarcolemma

D. Myosin

39. One gram of protein contains _____ calories.

A. 4

B. 7

C. 9

D. 11

40. Which of the following periodization cycles is used to plan and organize the overall training program?

A. Mesocycle

B. Microcycle

C. Macrocycle

D. Minicycle

41. Which of the following best describes a hook grip?

A. Thumb is placed underneath the middle and index fingers

B. Thumbs over the bar and fingers wrapped around the bar

C. The hands placed underneath the bar so the knuckles aim backward

D. Palms facing downwards with fingers intertwined

42. Which of these statements is not true about slow oxidative fibers (type I)?

A. They have a rich supply of mitochondria

B. They appear white in color

C. They are resistant to fatigue

D. They use aerobic respiration to generate ATP

43. Which of these muscles is responsible for straightening the leg at the knee?

A. The quadriceps femoris muscle

B. The hamstring muscles

C. The biceps femoris muscle

D. The iliopsoas muscle

44. Which of the following cells contribute to bone remodeling?

I. Osteoclasts

II. Osteoblasts

III. Osteocytes

A. I and III

B. I and II

C. II and III

D. I, II and III

45. Which of the following vitamins is considered toxic in excess amounts?

A. Vitamin C.

B. Vitamin B12

C. Vitamin B1

D. Vitamin A

46. What is the recommended minimum distance between the floor and the bottom of mirrors on the walls?

A. 18 inches (41cm)

B. 20 inches (51cm)

C. 22 inches (56cm)

D. 24 inches (60cm)

47. The process of combining mental and physical techniques to help an athlete replace a fear response to various cues with a relaxed response is referred to as?

A. Mental imagery

B. Optimal functioning

C. Systematic desensitization

D. Negative reinforcement

48. Which of the following relaxation techniques involves the athlete alternating between tensing and relaxing different muscle groups?

A. Progressive Muscle Relaxation (PMR)

B. Autogenic training

C. Deep breathing exercise

D. Guided imagery

49. Which of the following is a macronutrient?

A. Magnesium

B. Protein

C. Water

D. Vitamin E

50. What is the minimum recommended space between the ends of racks to provide room for spotters?

A. 1 foot (30cm)

B. 2 feet (61cm)

C. 3 feet (91cm)

D. 5 feet (152cm)

51. Which of these is not true about skeletal muscles?

A. The skeletal muscle is multinucleated

B. It is involuntary

C. The muscle fiber is made of actin and myosin

D. It is striated

52. Which of the following best describes the stretch-shortening cycle?

A. A rapid sequence of eccentric and concentric muscle contractions

B. The lengthening of a muscle during a static stretch

C. The transition between the eccentric and concentric phases of an exercise

D. The process of muscle fibers shortening during a concentric contraction

53. You are designing a training program for a 60-year-old female golfer; which of the following should be evaluated first?

A. Endurance

B. Medical history

C. Flexibility

D. Core strength.

54. Calisthenics is an example of a _____ of exercise.

A. Variable-resistance training method

B. Bodyweight training method

C. Nontraditional implement training method

D. Core stability and balance training method

55. The typical diet of a baseball player who weighs 200 pounds includes 300 grams of carbohydrates, 80 grams of protein, and 100 grams of fat each day. How much of his daily calorie consumption comes from fat, as a percentage?

A. 21%

B. 27%

C. 37%

D. 57%

56. Which of the following is not an important question to be considered when assessing facility design and layout?

A. How many athletes will use the facility?

B. What are the demographics of the athletes?

C. What are the training objectives for the athletes, coaches, and administration?

D. What is the color of the facility's walls?

57. Which of these is not a phase in the sprinting technique training?

A. Drive phase

B. Acceleration phase

C. Delivery phase

D. Recovery phase

58. Which of the following involves gradually increasing the difficulty of a strength training routine to continue promoting muscle growth and avoiding adaptation?

A. Circuit training

B. Progressive overload

C. Circuit training

D. Unilateral training

59. The following are ways alcohol impairs aerobic performance except?

A. Slowing down the citric acid cycle

B. Inhibiting gluconeogenesis

C. Raising lactate levels

D. Decreased cortisol levels

60. Which of these forms is incorrect in an athlete trying to perform the five-point body contact position while lying face up?

A. The head is securely positioned on the bench

B. The buttocks are evenly positioned on the bench or seat

C. The right foot is resting flat on the ground

D. Shoulders and head off the floor

61. What is the name of the phenomenon where an athlete loses their muscular endurance after a two-week vacation, despite months of training?

A. Detraining

B. Overtraining

C. Overreaching

D. Unloading

62. Which of the following triggers muscle contraction?

A. Acetylcholine

B. Calcium influx

C. ATP hydrolysis

D. All of the above

63. All these are metabolic consequences of the adaptations of muscle to endurance exercise except?

A. The slower use of glycogen and glucose in muscles

B. Increased reliance on fat oxidation

C. Increased lactate production during exercise

D. Increased number of mitochondria

64. Which of the following muscle properties is an athlete most likely trying to improve through the dumbbell curl performed with a light weight for 15 reps in one set?

A. Muscle endurance

B. Muscle strength

C. Power

D. Hypertrophy

65. Physiological adaptation to exercise involves which of the following?

I. Increased resting heart rate

II. Increased stroke volume

III. Decreased cardiac output

IV. Increased oxygen uptake

A. I, II, and III

B. I, III, and IV

C. II, and IV

D. I, III, and IV

66. All these are limitations of body weight training except?

A. They may become repetitive and boring over time

B. It may be difficult to isolate some specific muscle groups

C. They are not scalable

D. It may be difficult to achieve maximum strength gains

67. When an athlete is performing dumbbell exercises, where is the best place for the spotter to position his hands?

A. On the athlete's upper arms

B. On the athlete's elbow

C. Near the athlete's wrists at their forearms

D. Near the athlete's hips

68. Which of the following training protocols is likely to lead to the most significant improvement in muscular strength?

A. 5 sets of 5 reps

B. 1 set of 5 reps

C. 5 sets of 15 reps

D. 1 set of 15 reps

69. _____ is/are the functional unit of muscle cells

A. Sarcolemma

B. Sarcoplasm

C. Sarcomere

D. Epimysium

70. Which of these is a component of the emergency response plan?

A. Communication plan

B. Personnel and equipment roles and responsibilities

C. Training and exercises

D. All of the above are components of the emergency response plan

71. Which fuel source, when depleted, hinders marathon performance the most?

A. Glycogen

B. Triglycerides

C. Glucose

D. Creatine phosphate

72. How many ATPs are produced when one glucose molecule in the blood is degraded and broken down by the oxidative energy system?

A. 31

B. 38

C. 45

D. 47

73. When designing a new free weights facility, where in the room should you place the dumbbells?

A. Lined up along the wall

B. In the middle of the room

C. Near the cardiopulmonary training equipment

D. Right side of the room

74. Which of these is not a phase in the designing of a new strength and conditioning facility?

A. The pre-design phase

B. The construction phase

C. The conditioning phase

D. The design phase

75. _____ is responsible for pumping blood to the lungs where it becomes oxygenated.

A. The right atrium

B. The right ventricle

C. The left atrium

D. The left ventricle

76. Which of these activities places the most metabolic demand on the aerobic energy system?

A. Weight lifting

B. Soccer

C. Gymnastics

D. Swimming

77. Which of these muscle fibers are more resistant to fatigue?

A. Fast glycolytic fibers

B. Slow twitch fibers

C. Type IIa fibers

D. Fast-twitch fibers

78. What is the primary role of the hormone cortisol in exercise?

A. Promoting muscle growth

B. Increasing fat metabolism

C. Regulating blood sugar levels

D. Stimulating bone growth

79. In plyometric exercises, athletes who weigh more than 220 lbs. should not perform depth jumps from heights greater than _____.

A. 42 inches

B. 36 inches

C. 18 inches

D. 9 inches

80. In plyometric training, which phase involves the rapid transition between the eccentric and concentric phases of a movement?

A. Stretch-shortening cycle

B. Amortization phase

C. Concentric phase

D. Eccentric phase

81. Which of these energy systems does an athlete's body primarily depend on during a three-minute period in a wrestling match?

A. The glycolytic system

B. The phosphagen or ATP-CP

C. The oxidative/aerobic system

D. The lactic energy system

82. Which of these sequences of exercise would you recommend while instructing an athlete on exercise order during her training session?

A. Power clean, leg extensions, squats

B. Squats, leg extensions, power clean

C. Power clean, squats, leg extensions

D. Leg extensions, power clean, squats

83. Which of these muscle actions produces the greatest amount of muscle force?

A. Eccentric

B. Isometric

C. Concentric

D. Both B and C

84. A 21-year-old female college athlete began a strength and conditioning program 12 weeks ago. In the weeks following, she sees continuous gains in her strength. Which of the following most likely contributes to this change?

A. Improved neuromuscular efficiency

B. Increased mitochondria

C. Conversation of Type I to Type II muscle fibers

D. Muscular hypertrophy

85. Which of these validity testing methods is informal and non-quantitative?

A. Construct validity

B. Concurrent validity

C. Predictive validity

D. Face validity

86. During the late support phase of the sprint cycle, which movement helps to decelerate the backward rotation of the thigh?

A. Eccentric hip flexion

B. Eccentric plantar flexion

C. Concentric knee extension

D. Concentric plantar flexion

87. What phase in the design of the strength and conditioning facility involves creating detailed plans and specifications for the facility, including drawings, equipment lists, and detailed cost estimates?

A. Pre-design phase

B. Pre-operation phase

C. The design phase

D. Construction phase

88. As a coach, you noticed that one of your athletes is exhibiting signs of anorexia nervosa. What will be your best line of action?

A. Create a diet plan for the athlete

B. Put the athlete on leave

C. Refer the athlete to an eating disorder specialist

D. Request frequent weigh in

89. Which of the following exercise sessions results in the largest increase in serum HGH concentration?

A. Moderate-intensity aerobic exercise

B. High-intensity aerobic exercise

C. Moderate-intensity resistance exercise

D. High-intensity resistance exercise

90. What is the relative involvement of Type I and Type II muscle fibers in soccer?

A. Type I: High Involvement, Type II: Low Involvement

B. Type I: Low Involvement, Type II: High Involvement

C. Type I: High Involvement, Type II: High Involvement

D. Type I: Low Involvement, Type II: Low Involvement

91. Which of these is not a phase in the stretch-shortening cycle?

A. Isometric phase

B. Eccentric phase

C. Concentric phase

D. Amortization phase

92. Which of the following best describes the "SAID" principle in strength and conditioning?

A. Specific Adaptation to Imposed Demands

B. Sudden Activation of Intrinsic Dynamics

C. Systematic Approach to Individual Development

D. Standard Assessment of Isokinetic Devices

93. A 180 lb. baseball player has an average daily intake of 600g of carbohydrates, 140 g of fat, and 120 g of protein. What percent of his total calorie intake is protein?

A. 28%

B. 15%

C. 38%

D. 12%

94. Which of the following does not have a significant effect on flexibility?

A. Age

B. Joint structure

C. Dietary intake

D. Gender

95. Which of the following is an effect of heavy resistance exercise on cardiac output (CO)?

A. Increases CO rapidly

B. Decreases CO

C. Decreases CO rapidly

D. No significant change in CO

96. Which of these performance-enhancing substances is most likely to increase lean body mass?

A. Caffeine

B. Anabolic steroids

C. Ephedrine

D. Creatinine

97. Which of the following is NOT a component of the General Adaptation Syndrome (GAS)?

A. Alarm stage

B. Overreaching stage

C. Resistance stage

D. Exhaustion stage

98. The _____ muscle is commonly referred to as a "six-pack" in athletic individuals.

A. Pyramidalis

B. Rectus abdominis

C. External abdominal oblique

D. Internal abdominal oblique

99. Which of the following exercises exclusively targets the core?

A. Plank

B. Deadlift

C. Olympic lift

D. All of the above

100. The measure of the total amount of physical work performed during a workout session or over the course of an exercise program is referred to as_____?

A. Training intensity

B. Training volume

C. Training frequency

D. Training load

101. Which type of validity is considered the most accurate when assessing the quality of a test?

A. Content validity

B. Criterion-related validity

C. Construct validity

D. Face validity

102. Which type of muscle fibers are most resistant to fatigue?

A. Type I

B. Type IIa

C. Type IIb

D. Type IIx

103. In the context of resistance training, which of the following best defines the term "volume"?

A. The intensity of an exercise

B. The number of exercises performed

C. The total amount of weight lifted

D. The number of repetitions and sets

104. What are the minimum landing surface dimensions of a plyometric box?

A. 18 x 24 inches

B. 16 x 24 inches

C. 24 x 32 inches

D. 10 x 16 inches

105. Which of the following theories explains why some athletes react with excitement and anticipation when experiencing high levels of arousal, rather than with fear and anxiety?

A. Inverted-U Hypothesis

B. Optimal Functioning Theory

C. Catastrophe Theory

D. Reversal Theory

106. Which of the following exercises involves a first-class lever?

A. Standing heel raise

B. Triceps extension

C. Dumbbell biceps curl

D. Nodding a soccer ball

107. Which of the following is a small space between the presynaptic neuron and the postsynaptic cell?

A. Synaptic bulb

B. Dendrites

C. Axons

D. Synaptic cleft

108. Which of the following adaptations to training helps to reduce the acidic levels in the muscle?

A. Increased capillary density

B. Increased glycogen and fat stores

C. Increased removal of lactate

D. Increased stroke volume

109. What is the impact of recovery stages on training?

A. Delay the onset of physiological adaptations

B. Decrease the rate of recovery from exercise-induced fatigue

C. Improve the rate of adaptation to endurance training

D. Help athletes recover from exercise-induced fatigue and prevent overtraining

110. What type of training is muscular hypertrophy beneficial for?

A. Endurance training

B. Aerobic training

C. Strength and power training

D. None of the above

111. How does alcohol impair aerobic performance?

A. By increasing lactate levels

B. By increasing glucose production

C. By increasing oxygen uptake

D. By increasing muscle strength

112. All of these are reported adverse effects of creatine supplementation, except?

A. Muscle stiffness

B. Nausea

C. Weight loss

D. Increased muscle strains

113. Which of the following statements is not accurate about tire selection and setup for tire flips as part of the college football team's off-season conditioning program for an offensive lineman?

A. The tire should be taller than the athlete

B. The tread surface should be free from exposed metal

C. The exercise surface should be hard

D. The athlete should use a narrower tire

114. Which of the following is not one of the main objectives of sport psychology?

A. Determining psychological aspects through measurement

B. Studying the relationship between psychological variables and athletic performance

C. Increasing sales of sports equipment

D. Enhancing athletes' performance

115. Which of the following is the maximum daily intake that is unlikely to have a negative impact on health?

A. Tolerable Upper Intake Level (TUL)

B. Recommended Dietary Allowance (RDA)

C. Adequate Intake (AI)

D. Estimated Average Requirement (EAR)

116. What is the recommended fluid intake before exercise?

A. 10-12 ounces

B. 16-20 ounces

C. 5-7 ounces

D. 20-24 ounces

117. Which of the following is a characteristic of anorexia nervosa?

A. Compulsive overeating

B. Binge eating followed by purging

C. Craving and eating non-food items

D. Severe restriction of food intake

118. What type of motivation is most commonly associated with pursuing a professional sports career for financial gain?

A. Intrinsic motivation

B. Extrinsic motivation

C. Mental motivation

D. Group motivation

119. Which of these combinations of nutrients can help optimize bone density in the elderly population?

A. Vitamin B12 and Potassium

B. Vitamin C and iron

C. Calcium and Vitamin D

D. Magnesium and potassium

120. Which of the following statements is an incorrect execution of the deadlift exercise technique?

A. Keeping the back straight and tight throughout the lift

B. Bending the knees and lowering the hips to reach the bar

C. Allowing the bar to drift away from the body during the lift

D. Engaging the core muscles to maintain stability during the lift

121. What is the primary function of the Golgi tendon organ?

A. Muscle contraction

B. Inhibition of muscle contraction

C. Proprioception

D. Stretch reflex activation

122. Which of the following exercises is classified as a closed kinetic chain exercise?

A. Leg extension

B. Leg curl

C. Seated calf raise

D. Squat

123. Regarding a resistance training program, which is the ideal exercise to perform first during a training session?

A. Isolation exercise

B. Multi-joint exercise

C. Warm-up exercise

D. Cool-down exercise

124. A 35-year-old recreational athlete has been participating in a strength training program for the past year and has noticed an improvement in their bench press 1 repetition maximum (1RM). Which of the following adaptations is most likely responsible for the improvement in their 1RM?

A. Increased cross-sectional area of muscle fibers

B. Increased neural drive to muscle fibers

C. Increased activity of the muscle fibers' contractile proteins

D. Increased number of muscle fibers available for activation

125. Which of the following statements is most accurate about age?

A. Chronological age measures the number of years that have passed, while biological age is a measure of overall growth and development

B. Chronological age and biological age are the same thing and reflect the same stages of development

C. Biological age is a measure of the individual's weightlifting experience, while chronological age is a measure of maturity

D. Chronological age is a measure of maturity based on physical appearance, while biological age is a measure of maturity based on sexual development

126. The daily sodium recommendation is _____.

A. 1200 milligrams per day

B. 3400 milligrams per day

C. 4000 milligrams per day

D. 2300 milligrams per day

127. Which of these foods is a source of potassium?

A. Bananas

B. Pretzels

C. Flax seeds

D. White rice

128. Which of the following ways can an athlete increase their vitamin D?

A. Getting regular sun exposure

B. Eating more citrus fruits

C. Reducing their protein intake

D. Consuming more lentils

129. In adults, athletes taking more than 1,500 IU/day of vitamin E are at an increased risk of _____.

A. Scurvy

B. Osteoporosis

C. Muscle cramps

D. Hemorrhage

130. Which of the following is a way arginine improves muscle growth?

A. By increasing human growth hormone secretion

B. By reducing inflammation

C. By decreasing blood flow to the muscles

D. By inhibiting protein synthesis

131. Which of the following common supplements used by athletes promotes faster recovery after exercise?

A. Creatine

B. Beta-hydroxy-beta-methylbutyrate (HMB)

C. Betaine

D. Glutamine

132. Which of the following is an important role of iron supplements in exercise?

A. Improved endurance exercise performance

B. Increased muscle strength

C. Enhanced oxygen delivery to muscles

D. Reduced muscle damage and inflammation

133. Which of the following is a banned substance that is often used as a diuretic and masking agent to hide the use of other performance enhancing drugs?

A. Creatine

B. Caffeine

C. Nitric oxide

D. Furosemide

134. Which grip type is recommended for individuals with weak grip strength?

A. Hook grip

B. Closed grip

C. False grip

D. Alternated grip

135. Which of the following is a potential risk associated with the Valsalva maneuver?

A. Increased intra-abdominal pressure

B. Decreased blood pressure

C. Improved breathing efficiency

D. Reduced core stability

136. As a coach, which of the following is the most effective way to implement progressive overload in a resistance training program?

A. By increasing the rest times

B. By decreasing the intensity of exercises

C. By increasing the volume of training by adding more sets or reps

D. By maintaining the same weight and reps for each exercise

137. Which of the following statements is true about repetition ranges?

A. Low repetition ranges (1-5 reps) are associated with fast-twitch muscle fibers

B. High repetition ranges (8-15 reps) and heavy weight are used for muscular endurance

C. High repetition ranges (15-20+ reps) are associated with intermediate-twitch muscle fibers

D. Low repetition ranges (2-5 reps) with lighter weight are used for building muscle mass and strength

138. Which of the following is an example of a tempo recommendation?

A. 5 sets of 10 reps at 80% 1RM

B. 3 seconds eccentric, 0 seconds pause, 1 second concentric, 0 seconds pause

C. 3 sets of 12 reps with a 60-second rest interval between sets

D. 4 exercises targeting different muscle groups

139. Which of the following is a key element of the snatch lift?

A. The press

B. The clean

C. The jerk

D. The pull

140. During the snatch lift, at what point should the lifter accelerate and perform a triple extension of the knees, ankles, and hips?

A. Before grabbing the bar

B. When lifting the bar up past the chest

C. When the bar is past the knees

D. When standing on their toes

141. Which of the following is a major disadvantage of Olympic lifting?

A. Requires a significant amount of coaching time and attention

B. It is overly simplistic

C. It doesn't provide a full-body workout

D. It is not a popular form of exercise

142. How many major models of plyometric exercise are there?

A. 2

B. 3

C. 4

D. 5

143. Which muscle group is most commonly targeted in plyometric exercises?

A. Upper body

B. The core

C. Lower body

D. Full body

144. All of these are key factors in improving speed, except?

A. Stride frequency

B. Stride length

C. Vertical force

D. Muscle endurance

145. Which of the following factors can impact an athlete's recovery needs?

A. Age

B. Gender

C. Training experience

D. All of the above

146. Which of the following is the first step in a needs analysis?

A. The sport or activity being analyzed

B. The athlete's training history

C. The athlete's performance goals

D. The athlete's dietary habits

147. What type of information is typically collected during the assessment phase of a needs analysis?

A. Information about the athlete's training history

B. Information about the athlete's medical history

C. Information about the athlete's performance goals

D. All of the above

148. Which of the following is not typically included in a sport-specific needs analysis?

A. Assessment of the athlete's current physical condition

B. Evaluation of the athlete's mental readiness

C. Analysis of the athlete's cultural background

D. Examination of the demands of the sport or activity

149. In what way can the progression of unilateral exercises be modified to increase the training stimulus?

A. By decreasing the number of sets and reps

B. By increasing the rest periods between sets

C. By using heavier weights and lower reps

D. By incorporating balance and stability challenges

150. All of these are examples of a unilateral exercise, except?

A. Bench press

B. Single arm bicep curls

C. Split squat

D. Romanian deadlift

151. Which of the following methods of training involves holding the muscle in a static position to build strength?

A. Unilateral

B. Bilateral

C. Isometric

D. Plyometric

152. Which of these exercises should be performed first in a training session when considering the fatigability of muscles?

A. Low-intensity exercise

B. Single-joint accessory exercises

C. High-intensity exercise

D. It doesn't matter the order of priority

153. Which of the following exercises should be prioritized first during training?

A. Leg extensions

B. Bicep curls

C. Squats

D. Quadriceps extension

154. Which of the following is not a key component of the emergency response plan for a strength and conditioning facility?

A. Emergency medical services activation process

B. Contact information for primary, secondary, and tertiary emergency contacts

C. Exact location of the strength and conditioning center for emergency responders

D. A list of all equipment in the facility

155. In the event of a fire in a strength and conditioning facility, which of the following steps should be taken first?

A. Evacuate the building

B. Call 911 or the local emergency services number

C. Attempt to extinguish the fire

D. Notify the facility's management team

156. All these are key variables to monitor in agility, except?

A. Change-of-direction deficit

B. Acceleration

C. Ground contact time

D. Exit velocity

157. Which of the following best describes the difference between macronutrients and micronutrients?

A. Macronutrients are required in larger quantities than micronutrients

B. Micronutrients provide energy, while macronutrients do not

C. Macronutrients are essential, while micronutrients are non-essential

D. There is no difference between macronutrients and micronutrients

158. What is the first disciplinary measure taken for an athlete violating the facility's rules?

A. Dismissal from the facility for one day

B. Dismissal from the facility for one week

C. A verbal warning by a staff member

D. Permanent dismissal from the facility

159. Which of the following is not a disciplinary measure taken for violating the facility's rules?

A. Dismissal from the facility for one day

B. Dismissal from the facility for one week

C. Verbal abuse by a staff member

D. Dismissal from the facility for the remainder of the year

160. When developing a workout routine for a golfer who is 70-years-old, the first thing that should be taken into consideration is which of the following?

A. Upper body strength

B. Core strength

C. Flexibility

D. Medical history

161. During which phase of the periodization cycle is an athlete most likely to focus on developing maximum strength?

A. Hypertrophy phase

B. Strength phase

C. Power phase

D. Recovery phase

162. A soccer player is performing a push-up during a training session. Which type of lever occurs at the elbow joint during this exercise?

A. First class

B. Second class

C. Third class

D. Fourth class

163. In which plane of action does the abduction of the arms occur during the butterfly stroke in swimming?

A. Sagittal

B. Frontal

C. Transverse

D. Oblique

164. A weightlifter lifts a 60 kg barbell 1.5 m off the ground for 10 repetitions in 25 seconds. What is the power output?

A. 225 W

B. 353 W

C. 375 W

D. 450 W

165. Which of the following is a primary antagonist muscle group during the bench press exercise?

A. Biceps brachii

B. Triceps brachii

C. Latissimus dorsi

D. Pectoralis major

166. How does the patella contribute to the mechanical advantage of the quadriceps muscle group?

A. It decreases the length of the quadriceps tendons

B. It decreases the moment arm of the quadriceps tendon

C. It increases the amount of force generated by the quadriceps muscle group.

D. It maintains the angle of the patellar tendon to the tibial tuberosity.

167. Which of the following exercises primarily occurs in the frontal plane?

A. Lateral raises

B. Bicep curls

C. Tricep extensions

D. Shoulder presses

168. What should be the FIRST priority when incorporating agility drills into the conditioning program of a 15-year-old girl?

A. Building stamina

B. Building muscle mass

C. Developing proper technique

D. All of the above

169. Which of the following states of muscle length is associated with the greatest force production capability?

A. Shortened

B. Stretched

C. Contracted

D. Resting

170. Which of the following best describes the relationship between a motor unit and the number of muscle fibers it innervates?

A. A motor unit innervates many muscle fibers.

B. A motor unit innervates only a single muscle fiber

C. A motor unit does not innervate any muscle fibers

D. None of the above

171. What is the primary purpose of a dynamic warm-up?

A. To increase heart rate and blood flow

B. To improve flexibility and joint range of motion

C. To activate and mobilize the muscles

D. All of the above

172. Which muscles are worked in the glute bridge exercise?

A. Hamstrings

B. Calves

C. Glutes

D. Abs

173. Which of the following equipment is necessary to perform an upper body pushing exercise?

A. Dumbbells

B. A pull-up bar

C. A weight bench

D. A resistance band

174. How should the barbell be positioned for a high-bar Olympic squat?

A. Resting on the shoulders

B. Held in front of the body

C. Balanced on the hips

D. Balanced on the head

175. Which muscles are worked in the shoulder press exercise?

A. Chest, shoulders, and triceps

B. Biceps, back, and abs

C. Glutes, hamstrings, and quads

D. Shoulders and triceps

176. What is the proper form when performing a glute bridge?

A. Lie on your stomach and lift your legs and arms off the ground

B. Lie on your back with your knees bent and raise your hips toward the ceiling

C. Stand with your feet shoulder-width apart and bend your knees

D. Sit on a bench with a barbell at shoulder height and press it overhead

177. What skills are required for a Strength and Conditioning professional?

A. Administration and management only

B. Sport/exercise science only

C. Coaching and teaching only

D. A combination of sport/exercise science, administration, management, teaching, and coaching skills

178. What is the most important aspect of facility design and layout for strength and conditioning coaches?

A. The demographics of the athletes

B. The number of athletes who will use the facility

C. The equipment that needs to be repaired or modified

D. The training objectives for the athletes, coaches, and administration

179. A gymnast mentally rehearses a difficult routine before attempting it on the balance beam. What is this athlete engaging in?

A. Mental imagery

B. Extreme exercise

C. Mind psychoanalysis

D. All of the above

180. What is the main difference between linear periodization and undulating periodization?

A. In linear periodization, training volume and intensity are alternated on a daily or weekly basis, while in undulating periodization, they are gradually increased over time

B. In linear periodization, training volume and intensity are gradually increased over time, while in undulating periodization, they are alternated on a daily or weekly basis

C. Linear periodization focuses on endurance training, while undulating periodization focuses on strength training

D. Undulating periodization is only used in power and strength sports, while linear periodization is used in all sports

181. Which periodization model begins with high intensity and low volume and gradually decreases the intensity while increasing the volume over time?

A. Linear periodization

B. Block periodization

C. Undulating periodization

D. Reverse periodization

182. What is informed consent in sports?

A. A process where participants are not informed of the risks of participation

B. A process where risks are explained to participants and they make an uninformed decision to participate

C. A process where risks are explained to participants and they make an informed decision to participate

D. A process where participants are not required to make a decision to participate

183. Which energy system would primarily supply ATP for short, high-intensity activities such as weightlifting or sprinting?

A. The phosphagen energy system

B. The glycolytic energy system

C. The oxidative energy system

D. The creatine kinase energy system

184. For which of the following activities would the phosphagen energy system be the primary source of ATP?

A. Running a 100-meter dash

B. Running a 400-meter dash

C. Running a 1600-meter race

D. Running a marathon

185. A female gymnast is unable to perform a complicated routine during a competition. Which of the following factors is most likely to have limited her performance?

A. Inadequate warm-up

B. Depleted muscle glycogen

C. Dehydration

D. Low oxygen levels in the blood

186. Which of the following factors will primarily determine the dominant energy system used during a weightlifting session?

A. Exercise intensity and athlete's age

B. Exercise duration and athlete's age

C. Exercise intensity and exercise duration

D. Exercise intensity and athlete's training status

187. Which of the following factors does NOT affect the recovery time needed for an athlete after a high-intensity interval training session?

A. The duration of the exercise session

B. The athlete's age

C. The intensity of the exercise session

D. The athlete's gender

188. What is a common side effect of taking iron supplements at doses greater than 45 mg/day?

A. Increased muscle mass

B. Galactorrhea

C. Lowered lactate concentration

D. Gastric upset

189. Which of the following sports would benefit the most from caffeine supplementation?

A. Weightlifting

B. Marathon running

C. Soccer

D. Swimming

190. What is the name of the instrument used to measure blood pressure?

A. Sphygmomanometer

B. Otoscope

C. Stethoscope

D. Ophthalmoscope

191. Which of the following is a marker of overreaching during exercise training?

A. Increased resting heart rate

B. Increased muscle strength

C. Increased total testosterone concentration

D. Decreased lactate threshold

192. When performing a bicep curl, which of the following is a common mistake?

A. Rapidly swinging the weight to generate momentum

B. Contracting the triceps throughout the movement

C. Fully extending the elbows at the bottom of the movement

D. Keeping the wrists in a neutral position

193. How can understanding organizational trends and best practices in strength and conditioning help a strength and conditioning specialist?

A. Stay current with the latest research

B. Implement best practices in their program

C. Provide better training to athletes

D. All of the above

194. Why is communicating the results an important step in sports evaluation and interpretation?

A. To identify patterns and trends in data using statistical methods

B. To make sense of data and determine implications for the athlete's training and recovery

C. To share the results with the appropriate stakeholders

D. To collect information from monitoring protocols and procedures

195. What is content validity in sports analysis used for?

A. To ensure that a test covers the entire range of the construct or variable being measured

B. To determine the ability of a test to predict future performance in a sport

C. To differentiate between two distinct constructs

D. To determine the relationship between a test and a criterion measure

196. Which of the following is the purpose of retest reliability?

A. To compare two different versions of the same test

B. To measure the consistency of scores across raters or test forms

C. To assess the consistency of test results over time

D. To determine the relationship between a test and another measure that is currently in use

197. Which of the following exercises is a lower body pushing exercise that targets the quadriceps, glutes, and lower back muscles?

A. Bench press

B. Shoulder press

C. Deadlift

D. High-bar Olympic squat

198. A female bodybuilder wants to increase her muscle mass and decrease body fat. She currently consumes 2200 kilocalories per day, consisting of 25% fat, 30% protein, and 45% carbohydrate. Which of the following guidelines will be MOST important to achieve her goal?

A. Decrease carbohydrate, increase fat, and reduce protein

B. Increase carbohydrate, decrease fat, and maintain protein

C. Maintain current proportions but increase overall calorie intake

D. Decrease overall calorie intake, increase protein, and decrease fat

199. Which of the following tests is most appropriate for assessing a male soccer player's agility?

A. 1 RM squat

B. 20-meter sprint

C. T-test

D. Standing long jump

200. You are observing a group of weightlifters performing the squat. Which of the following is a common error?

A. Leaning too far forward during the descent

B. Keeping the feet parallel to each other

C. Fully extending the knees at the top of the movement

D. Feet remaining flat on the ground

201. What is the recommended rest interval between sets for strength and power training to optimize neuromuscular recovery?

A. 30-60 seconds

B. 1-2 minutes

C. 2-5 minutes

D. 5-10 minutes

202. Which of the following exercises primarily targets the latissimus dorsi muscle?

A. Pull-up

B. Push-up

C. Bench press

D. Seated row

203. Which exercises primarily target the chest muscles?

I. Push-ups

II. Bicep curls

III. Lunges

IV. Squats

A. I only

B. II only

C. I and II only

D. I and IV only

204. Which of the following are benefits of high-intensity interval training (HIIT)?

I. Improves cardiovascular fitness

II. Burns more calories than steady-state cardio

III. Increases muscle mass

IV. Can be completed in a short amount of time

A. I and II only

B. II and III only

C. I, II, and IV only

D. I, III, and IV only

205. Which of the following is the most appropriate progression of plyometric exercises for a beginner?

A. Depth jumps → single-leg hops → box jumps

B. Box jumps → single-leg hops → depth jumps

C. Jumps in place → box jumps → depth jumps

D. Depth jumps → box jumps → jumps in place

206. What is the main function of the rotator cuff muscles?

A. To rotate the arm at the shoulder joint

B. To stabilize the shoulder joint

C. To adduct the arm at the shoulder joint

D. To flex the arm at the elbow joint

207. A basketball player is performing a hang clean during their training. As the athlete transitions from the second pull to the catch phase, they find it difficult to fully extend their hips and ankles, resulting in a less than optimal catch position. What should the athlete do in this situation?

A. Complete the lift and reset for the next repetition

B. Use more arm strength to pull the bar to a higher position

C. Quickly drop the bar and step back from the lifting platform

D. Pause and work on improving hip and ankle mobility before attempting the next repetition

208. What is the primary function of the abdominal muscles during a squat?

A. Flexion of the spine

B. Stabilization of the spine

C. Extension of the spine

D. Lateral flexion of the spine

209. In a resistance training program, what does the term "rest interval" refer to?

A. The time between sets of an exercise

B. The time between individual repetitions within a set

C. The time between different exercises in a workout

D. The time between workouts

210. When performing a barbell overhead press, what position should your hands be in?

A. Pronated grip with both palms facing down

B. Neutral grip with palms facing each other

C. Supinated grip with both palms facing up

D. Alternated grip with one hand overhand and one hand underhand

211. How does autogenic training differ from progressive muscle relaxation?

A. Autogenic training involves focusing on your breathing, while progressive muscle relaxation involves alternating tensing and relaxing different muscle groups

B. Autogenic training replaces the muscle relaxation cycle with a focus on feelings of warmth and heaviness, while progressive muscle relaxation involves focusing on your breathing

C. Autogenic training involves replacing the muscle relaxation cycle with a focus on feelings of warmth and heaviness, while progressive muscle relaxation involves alternating tensing and relaxing different muscle groups

D. None of the above

212. Which of the following best describes the Valsalva maneuver?

A. Inhaling and exhaling rapidly during exercise to increase oxygen delivery

B. Holding your breath and bearing down to increase intra-abdominal pressure during heavy lifting

C. Breathing deeply and slowly to relax the body and reduce stress

D. None of the above

213. What is the estimated age-predicted maximum heart rate of a 25-year-old female who is 5'6" tall and weighs 130 lbs. with a resting heart rate of 65 beats per minute?

A. 180

B. 195

C. 205

D. 220

214. Which body part enhances the performance of the quadriceps muscle group by keeping the tendon away from the center of rotation at the knee?

A. The ankle

B. The hip

C. The knee cap (patella)

D. The shoulder

215. What is the anatomical position of the human body?

A. Lying down with arms at the sides

B. Standing upright with arms at the sides and facing forward

C. Sitting with legs crossed

D. Standing with arms crossed

216. What is the final portion of the clean and jerk lift called?

A. The clean

B. The jerk

C. The pull

D. The press

217. Which of the following physiological adaptations can delay muscle fatigue?

A. Decreased stroke volume

B. Decreased hemoglobin levels

C. Increased capillary density

D. Increased oxygen uptake

218. What is the effect of training on slow-twitch muscle fibers?

A. Increased anaerobic enzymes for glycolysis

B. Increased creatine phosphate stores

C. Increased mitochondrial density

D. Increased removal of lactate

219. An athlete's estimated one-rep max for the squat is 300 pounds. What is the appropriate training load for the client if the program calls for 75% of their one-rep max?

A. 210 pounds

B. 225 pounds

C. 250 pounds

D. 275 pounds

220. A client performs a set of 8 repetitions of a standing barbell curl with a weight of 80 pounds. What is the estimated one-rep max for the client based on the Brzycki formula?

A. 100 pounds

B. 110 pounds

C. 120 pounds

D. 130 pounds

Test 1 Answers and Explanations

1. (B) Larynx.

The larynx, also called the voice box, is a hollow tube that allows air to pass from the pharynx into the trachea. It is also responsible for the generation of sounds for speech. The pharynx, trachea, and epiglottis are all important organs in the respiratory system but they are not directly responsible for generating sounds for speech.

2. (C) Muscle spindles.

Muscle spindles are also called stretch detectors, and they detect changes in the length of a muscle. When a muscle is stretched or lengthened, the muscle spindle is also stretched, which activates the sensory neurons to send signals to the spinal cord and brain. The axon, dendrites, and synaptic cleft are components of neurons.

3. (A) Hematopoiesis.

Hematopoiesis is the process in which new blood cells (red blood cells, white blood cells, and platelets) are produced in the bone marrow. Leukopoiesis, erythropoiesis, and thrombopoiesis are all subtypes of hematopoiesis that specifically refer to the production of white blood cells, red blood cells, and platelets, respectively.

4. (C) 1:20.

A common recommendation for the coach-to-athlete ratio in colleges is 1:20. Typically, ratios between 1:15 and 1:20 are accepted. This is to allow the coach to provide individual attention and guidance to participants while also maintaining a safe and efficient training environment.

5. (B) Acetylcholine.

Acetylcholine is a neurotransmitter that is released by the motor neuron at the neuromuscular junction. It plays a huge role in muscle contraction. It does this by binding to receptors on the muscle fiber, leading to the depolarization of the muscle cell membrane and the initiation of an action potential, which ultimately leads to muscle contraction. Although troponin is involved in muscle contraction, it is not found at the neuromuscular junction. Acetylcholinesterase is an enzyme that breaks down acetylcholine, which stops contraction, while creatine phosphate is a molecule that provides energy for muscle contraction.

6. (C) Mediastinum.

The left and right lungs are separated by a compartment called the mediastinum. The diaphragm is a dome-shaped muscle that separates the thoracic cavity from the abdominal cavity. The pleural cavity is the space between the two layers of the pleural membrane, which surrounds each lung.

7. (B) Increased maximal heart rate.

in older adults, most physiological phenomena decrease. As such, heart rate, cardiac output, and maximal stroke volume are typically reduced. Therefore, an increase in maximal heart rate is not a physiological change that typically occurs with aging.

8. (C) Gymnastics.

Gymnastics is typically considered to be an advantage for teenage girls over teenage boys. This is because the sport emphasizes flexibility and agility, which comes more naturally to girls. However, keep in mind that both genders can participate in gymnastics. Boys, on the other hand, tend to excel in sports that require more raw strength and power, such as football and weightlifting. For basketball, there is no inherent advantage for one gender over the other.

9. (B) Acetylcholine is released.

The release of acetylcholine is required for muscle contraction to occur. All other factors such as calcium being pumped back into the sarcoplasmic reticulum, depleted ATP stores, and muscle cells being fatigued can cause the human muscle to stop contracting.

10. (B) Muscle glycogen.

For light marathons, muscle glycogen is the most probable limiting factor, followed by liver glycogen and fat stores.

11. (B) This type of reaction breaks down energy-storing molecules.

Anabolic reactions are a type of metabolic reaction that build complex molecules from simpler ones. Catabolic reactions break down complex molecules into simpler ones and usually release energy. Respiration is a catabolic reaction and involves the breakdown of glucose molecules to release energy in the form of ATP.

12. (D) This energy system is instantaneously available.

The only correct statement is option D. This is because the phosphagen system is characterized by its very rapid rate of ATP production, making it an instantaneous source of energy for the body. The phosphagen system is not oxygen dependent as it is an anaerobic energy system. It also uses high-energy phosphates, such as creatine phosphate, to rapidly resynthesize ATP and not carbohydrates.

13. (A) Axons.

The correct option is A. Nerve fibers that carry signals from the spinal cord to effector organs are referred to as axons. Dendrites are nerve fibers that receive signals from other cells. Muscle spindles detect changes in the length of a muscle. The synaptic cleft is a small space between the presynaptic neuron and the postsynaptic cell.

14. (B) 60-80 beats/min.

The normal heartbeat of an adult is 60-80 beats per minute.

15. (B) Lungs.

The correct answer is the lungs. The mediastinum houses the heart and other important structures like the blood vessels, esophagus, thymus, and lymph nodes. However, the lungs are not located in the mediastinum; they are situated in the thoracic cavity outside of the mediastinum.

16. (B) Promoting protein synthesis.

Promoting protein synthesis is a key mechanism responsible for the increase in muscle size and strength during strength training. While other factors such as increasing aerobic metabolism, increasing muscle fiber activation, and increased ATP storage can contribute to exercise performance and energy production, they are not the primary drivers of muscle growth and strength increases during strength training.

17. (C) Conducting electrical impulses

In the heart's conduction system, you'll find specialized muscle fibers called Purkinje fibers. Their primary responsibility during each heartbeat is to rapidly transmit electrical impulses from the atrioventricular node to the ventricles. This ensures that the heart muscle contracts in a coordinated and effective manner, necessary for the efficient pumping of blood throughout the body.

18. (A) Plank.

The plank is an example of an isometric exercise, which involves maintaining a static muscle contraction without any visible change in muscle length or joint movement. Isometric exercises help develop muscular endurance and stability.

19. (A) Perimysium.

The correct answer is A. The fascicles are bundles of skeletal muscle fibers that are surrounded by the perimysium. The endomysium surrounds a single muscle fiber, while the epimysium surrounds the collection of fascicles that comprise a single muscle.

20. (C) Phosphagen.

The phosphagen system uses creatine phosphate (CP) to rapidly produce ATP for high-intensity, short-duration activities, such as sprinting or lifting heavy weights.

21. (A) To provide energy for physical activity.

The primary role of carbohydrates in an athlete's diet is to provide energy for physical activity. Carbohydrates are the body's preferred source of fuel, especially during high-intensity and endurance activities.

22. (B) The principle of segmental interaction.

The correct option is B. The principle of segmental interaction states that energy in a system of linked bodies can be transferred across body segments and joints. This principle is a fundamental concept in biomechanics, and it highlights the importance of understanding how forces and movements are transmitted throughout the body during human movement.

23. (A) 1:3 to 1:5.

The ideal work-rest ratio for a system powered by the fast glycolytic energy system is generally considered to be around 1:3 to 1:5. This means that for every one unit of work, the athlete should rest for three to five units of time. This allows for sufficient time for the energy system to recover and replenish its stores of ATP.

24. (A) Inverted-U theory

The correct answer is the inverted-U theory. Inverted-U theory states that arousal helps performance up to a certain point, but if arousal goes beyond that point, it can start to hurt performance.

25. (C) I only.

The only correct statement is I because type IIx fibers are more prone to fatigue than type I. Statement II is wrong because Type IIx fibers have a poor supply of blood capillaries. Statement III is incorrect because competitive swimmers usually have high amounts of type I fibers, not type II. Statement IV is incorrect because Type IIa uses aerobic respiration to generate ATP.

26. (B) Forceful exhalation against a closed glottis

The Valsalva maneuver involves taking a deep breath and forcefully exhaling against a closed glottis, which helps to stabilize the trunk during heavy lifting.

27. (C) Smooth muscle.

Smooth muscle is not striated. It has a smooth and non-striated appearance under the microscope. However, cardiac and skeletal muscles are striated.

28. (A) Sarcolemma.

The plasma membrane of a muscle fiber is called the sarcolemma. The sarcoplasmic reticulum is a specialized type of endoplasmic reticulum found in muscle cells that is responsible for storing and releasing calcium ions for muscle contraction. The perimysium and epimysium are both layers of connective tissue that surround the muscle fibers.

29. (C) Sternocleidomastoid.

The muscle found in the neck is the sternocleidomastoid muscle. The sternocleidomastoid muscle is responsible for rotating and tilting the head, and also helps with flexion of the neck. The trapezius muscle is a large muscle that spans the back and neck. The pectoralis major muscle is found in the chest. The rectus abdominis muscle is found in the abdomen.

30. (A) Isotonic exercise.

Isotonic exercise involves movements with a constant resistance throughout the range of motion, often characterized by high-resistance, low-repetition activities. This type of exercise can be performed using free weights, weight machines, or resistance bands.

31. (B) Endurance training.

Endurance training targets aerobic metabolism and improves fatigue resistance. Strength training, on the other hand, targets muscle strength and size. Flexibility training focuses on improving joint mobility and range of motion. Power training can help to improve explosive power and athletic performance.

32. (B) 20-35%

The recommended daily intake of dietary fat for athletes is 20-35% of total calories to ensure adequate energy, essential fatty acids, and fat-soluble vitamin absorption.

33. (A) The process of replacing an old bone with a new bone.

Bone remodeling is the process through which the skeletal structure of the body is maintained by constantly breaking down and replacing old bone with new bone. It involves the action of osteoclasts, which break down old bone tissue, and osteoblasts, which form new bone tissue.

34. (D) All of the above.

All of the above factors can affect how the neuromuscular system adapts to exercise.

35. (D) The principle of force-motion.

The principle of force-motion, also known as Newton's First Law of Motion or the principle of inertia, states that before motion can occur, some forces must act first. In other words, this means that an object at rest will remain at rest unless acted upon by an external force.

36. (C) Quadriceps.

The agonist muscles during a barbell squat are the quadriceps. The transverse abdominis, internal oblique, and rectus abdominis are not agonist muscles during a barbell squat, as they are not primarily responsible for creating the movement. However, these muscles may play a supportive role in maintaining proper form and stability during the exercise.

37. (A) Mitochondria.

Fatty acid oxidation occurs in the mitochondria of the cell.

38. (D) Myosin.

The thick structural protein found inside the sarcomere is called myosin. Actin is also a structural protein found inside the sarcomere, but it is thin. Myosin and actin are the two main proteins responsible for muscle contraction in skeletal and cardiac muscle.

39. (A) 4.

One gram of protein contains approximately 4 calories.

40. (C) Macrocycle.

The macrocycle is the longest cycle, typically lasting several months to a year, and is used to plan and organize the overall training program. It usually covers the entire training season, which can be several months to a year or more and is typically divided into multiple training phases.

41. (A) Thumb is placed underneath the middle and index fingers.

A hook grip is a weightlifting grip technique in which the thumb is placed underneath the middle and index fingers, and the fingers are wrapped around the bar.

42. (B) They appear white in color.

Option B is incorrect. Type I fibers are often referred to as "red fibers" because they have a high content of myoglobin, a protein that binds oxygen in muscle cells. This gives them a darker, red color compared to Type II fibers, which are often called "white fibers" due to their lower myoglobin content and paler appearance.

43. (A). The quadriceps femoris muscle.

The quadriceps femoris muscle, located in the thigh, is responsible for straightening the leg at the knee. In contrast, the hamstring muscles flex the knee.

44. (D) I, II, and III.

All three cells—osteoclasts, osteoblasts, and osteocytes contribute to bone remodeling. Osteoclasts break down bone tissue. Osteoblasts are responsible for forming new bone tissue. Osteocytes help to maintain bone tissue and regulate the activity of osteoblasts and osteoclasts.

45. (D) Vitamin A.

Fat-soluble vitamins like vitamins A, D, E, and K can be stored in the liver and fatty tissues. Hence, when consumed in excess, they can accumulate, leading to toxicity. Vitamin A can lead to toxic levels in the body, resulting in hypervitaminosis. Hence, option D is correct.

46. (B) 20 inches (51cm)

Mirrors should be positioned at least 6 inches away from equipment and 20 inches above the floor to avoid damage from dropped weights or plates.

47. (C) Systematic desensitization.

The process of combining mental and physical techniques to help an athlete replace a fear response to various cues with a relaxed response is referred to as systematic desensitization.

48. (A) Progressive Muscle Relaxation (PMR).

Progressive Muscle Relaxation (PMR) is a technique that involves a series of tensing and relaxing exercises that are designed to promote physical and mental relaxation by reducing muscle tension and calming the mind.

49. (B) Protein.

Protein is a macronutrient. Macronutrients are nutrients that the body needs in large amounts to maintain normal body functions and provide energy. The three main macronutrients are protein, carbohydrates, and fats.

50. (C) 3 feet (91cm).

Racks and platforms should be spaced 3-4 feet (0.9-1.2 m) apart to avoid injury in case of a fall.

51. (B) It is involuntary.

The skeletal muscle is multinucleated, striated, and voluntary. Hence, the statement "it is involuntary" is incorrect.

52. (A) A rapid sequence of eccentric and concentric muscle contractions.

The stretch-shortening cycle describes a rapid sequence of eccentric and concentric muscle contractions, which can enhance force production and improve performance in tasks such as jumping, sprinting, and throwing.

53. (B) Medical history.

Before designing a training program for a 60-year-old female golfer, it is important to evaluate her medical history first. This would allow you to get valuable information on any pre-existing medical conditions, past injuries, and medications that may affect her ability to exercise safely and effectively.

54. (B) Bodyweight training method.

Calisthenics are an example of a bodyweight training method of exercise. This type of training uses the weight of the body as the resistance for exercises, rather than external weights or equipment.

55. (C) 37%.

1 gram of fat= 9 Kcal

1 gram of protein= 4 Kcal

1 gram of carbohydrate= 4 Kcal

First, calculate the total kilocalories from each macronutrient:

Total kilocalories from fat: 100g fat x 9 kcal/g = 900 kcal

Total kilocalories from protein: 80g protein x 4 kcal/g = 320 kcal

Total kilocalories from carbohydrate: 300g carbohydrate x 4 kcal/g = 1200 kcal

Next, add up the kilocalories from each macronutrient to get the total kilocalorie.

Total kilocalories = 900 kcal (from fat) + 320 kcal (from protein) + 1200 kcal (from   carbohydrate) = 2420 kcal

Hence, the percentage of kilocalories from fat = (900 kcal / 2420 kcal) x 100% = 37.2%.

56. (D) What is the color of the facility's walls?

The color of the facility's walls is not an important question to be considered when assessing facility design and layout. This is because the color of the facility's walls is not directly related to the functionality of the space.

57. (C) Delivery phase.

The delivery phase is not a phase in the sprinting technique training. Sprinting technique training can be divided into five categories: starting, acceleration, drive phase, recovery phase, and deceleration.

58. (B) Progressive overload.

Progressive overload involves gradually increasing the difficulty of a strength training routine to continue promoting muscle growth and avoiding adaptation.

59. (D) Decreased cortisol levels.

Decreased cortisol levels are not a way that alcohol impairs aerobic performance. Alcohol impairs aerobic performance by slowing the citric acid cycle, inhibiting gluconeogenesis, and raising lactate levels.

60. (D) Shoulders and head off the floor.

Shoulders and head off the floor are the incorrect form in an athlete trying to perform the five-point body contact position while lying face up. Having the shoulders and head off the floor can lead to improper alignment and an increased risk of injury.

61. (A) Detraining.

Detraining is the process of losing physical fitness and performance gains due to a reduction or break in training. This can occur when an athlete takes a break from training or reduces the intensity, duration, or frequency of their training.

62. (D) All of the above.

All the options are necessary for muscle contraction. Acetylcholine is the neurotransmitter that stimulates muscle contraction, and calcium influx is required for the initiation of muscle contraction. ATP hydrolysis provides the energy necessary for the muscle fibers to contract.

63. (C) Increased lactate production during exercise.

Increased lactate production during exercise is not a metabolic consequence of the adaptations of muscle to endurance exercise. This is because there is less lactate production during endurance exercise, as endurance training is associated with a reduced reliance on glycolysis and lactate production, and an increased reliance on fat oxidation for energy production.

64. (A) Muscle endurance.

The athlete is most likely trying to improve their muscle endurance by performing dumbbell curls with a light weight for 15 reps in one set. To improve muscle endurance, an athlete typically performs a high number of repetitions (such as 12 or more) with a relatively light weight, as in the case of the dumbbell curl described.

65. (C) II and IV.

Some physiological adaptations that occur during training include decreased resting heart rate, increased stroke volume, increased cardiac output, and increased oxygen uptake. Hence, only options II and IV are correct.

66. (C) They are not scalable.

Option C is wrong because bodyweight training can be easily scalable by adjusting the intensity, volume, and difficulty of the exercises, making it suitable for all fitness levels.

67. (C) Near the athlete's wrists at their forearms.

When spotting dumbbell exercises, it is crucial to spot close to the dumbbells or, in some cases, to spot the dumbbell itself. Hence, spotting near the athlete's wrists at their forearms is a safer technique.

68. (A) 5 sets of 5 reps.

The training protocol that is likely to lead to the most significant improvement in muscular strength is "5 sets of 5 reps". This protocol is commonly known as the "5x5" training program and is a popular strength training method used by athletes, powerlifters, and bodybuilders. The other training protocols listed in the question (1 set of 5 reps, 5 sets of 15 reps, and 1 set of 15 reps) are more suited for other training goals, such as muscular endurance (higher reps per set).

69. (C) Sarcomere.

The functional unit of a muscle cell is a "sarcomere." A sarcomere is the basic structural and functional unit of striated muscle, which includes skeletal and cardiac muscle.

70. (D). All of the above are components of the emergency response plan.

All of the components listed—emergency procedures and protocols, communication plan, personnel and equipment roles and responsibilities, and training and exercises—are typically considered essential for an effective emergency response plan.

71. (A) Glycogen.

The answer is glycogen. When glycogen stores become depleted, it can hinder marathon performance the most as the body relies more on fat as a fuel source. Triglycerides and glucose can also be used as fuel sources; however, they are not as readily available as glycogen.

72. (B) 38.

The degradation of one blood glucose molecule via the oxidative energy system produces approximately 38 ATP molecules.

73. (A) Lined up along the wall.

Placing the dumbbells along the wall provides enough space for free movement in the center of the room while keeping the weights easily accessible and visible to the users. If the dumbbells are placed in the middle of the room or near the cardiopulmonary training equipment, they can create congestion and safety hazards, and could limit the usable space for other exercises. Similarly, placing the dumbbells on the right side of the room could lead to uneven weight distribution and could limit the space available for other gym users.

74. (C) The conditioning phase.

Option C is incorrect. The four phases in designing a new strength and conditioning facility include the pre-design phase, design phase, construction phase, and pre-operation phase. The conditioning phase is not a phase in designing a new strength and conditioning facility.

75. (B) The right ventricle.

In the heart's cycle, deoxygenated blood returns to the heart and enters the right atrium. It then passes to the right ventricle, which pumps the blood to the lungs via the pulmonary arteries. In the lungs, the blood picks up oxygen and releases carbon dioxide, a process known as gas exchange. The oxygenated blood then returns to the heart, entering the left atrium, and then the left ventricle, which pumps the oxygen-rich blood to the rest of the body.

76. (D) Swimming.

Swimming places the most metabolic demand on the aerobic energy system. Soccer and gymnastics also use the aerobic energy system; however, they rely heavily on the anaerobic energy system for short bursts of high-intensity activity. Weight lifting is mainly an anaerobic activity that relies on the ATP-PC and glycolytic energy systems.

77. (B) Slow-twitch fibers.

Slow-twitch fibers, also known as Type I fibers, are more resistant to fatigue than other types of muscle fibers. This makes them ideal for activities like long-distance running, cycling, and other endurance sports.

78. C) Regulating blood sugar levels.

Cortisol, a catabolic hormone, is released during exercise to help maintain blood sugar levels by promoting the breakdown of proteins, fats, and carbohydrates for energy.

79. (C) 18 inches.

For athletes who weigh over 220 pounds, the height of the depth jump box should be 18 inches or less.

80. (B) Amortization phase.

The amortization phase in plyometric training is the brief transition period between the eccentric (muscle lengthening) and concentric (muscle shortening) phases of a movement, during which the muscle stores elastic energy to be released in the subsequent concentric phase.

81. (B) The phosphagen or ATP-CP energy system.

During a three-minute period in a wrestling match, an athlete's body primarily depends on the phosphagen or ATP-CP energy system. This system provides energy for short, high-intensity bursts of activity, such as the explosive movements required in wrestling.

82. (C) Power clean, squats, leg extensions.

The best option is C. Power clean, which is a multi-joint exercise, should be performed first, as it requires a high level of skill and power. Then, squats, which targets multiple muscle groups, including the quads, hamstrings, glutes, and core, and should be performed second. Finally, leg extensions should be performed last, as it is less complex and requires less skill and power compared to the power clean and squats.

83. (C) Concentric.

Concentric muscle actions generally produce the greatest amount of muscle force compared to eccentric and isometric muscle actions.

84. (A) Improved neuromuscular efficiency.

The most likely contributor to the continuous gains in strength seen by a 21-year-old female college athlete in the weeks following her strength and conditioning program is improved neuromuscular efficiency. While increases in mitochondrial density, muscle fiber type conversion, and muscular hypertrophy can all contribute to improvements in strength and athletic performance over time, these adaptations typically take longer to develop and are less likely to account for the initial gains seen in the early stages of a strength and conditioning program.

85. (D) Face validity.

Face validity refers to the perceived accuracy of a test or test item by the athlete and other casual observers. The evaluation of face validity is typically informal and non-quantitative.

86. (A) Eccentric hip flexion.

The eccentric hip flexion decelerates the backward rotation of the thigh.

87. (D) Construction phase.

The construction phase involves creating detailed plans and specifications for the facility, including drawings, equipment lists, and detailed cost estimates.

88. (C) Refer the athlete to an eating disorder specialist.

If you suspect that one of your athletes is exhibiting signs of anorexia nervosa, referring the athlete to an eating disorder specialist would be the best line of action as a coach.

89. (D) High-intensity resistance exercise.

High-intensity resistance exercise is the exercise session that results in the largest increase in serum HGH (human growth hormone) concentration.

90. (C) Type I: High involvement, Type II: High involvement.

In soccer, Type I (slow-twitch) and Type II (fast-twitch) muscle fibers are both involved to a high degree.

91. (A) Isometric phase.

The isometric phase is not a phase in the stretch-shortening cycle (SSC). The three phases of the SSC include the eccentric phase, amortization phase, and concentric phase.

92. (A) Specific Adaptation to Imposed Demands (SAID)

The SAID principle stands for Specific Adaptation to Imposed Demands, emphasizing that the body adapts specifically to the demands placed on it, making it essential to design training programs that target specific goals.

93. (D) 12%.

1 gram of fat= 9 Kcal

1 gram of protein= 4 Kcal

1 gram of Carbohydrate= 4 Kcal

Carbohydrates: 600g x 4 calories/gram = 2400 calories

Fat: 140g x 9 calories/gram = 1260 calories

Protein: 120g x 4 calories/gram = 480 calories

Total calories = 2400 + 1260 + 480 = 4140 calories

Percentage of calories from protein = (calories from protein/total calories) x 100% = (480/4140) x 100% = 11.59%

Approximately 12%.

94. (C) Dietary intake.

Dietary intake has the least significant effect on flexibility. Factors that can affect flexibility include age, joint structure, and gender.

95. (A) Increases CO rapidly.

During heavy resistance exercise, there is typically an initial increase in cardiac output (CO) in response to the increased oxygen demand by the muscles.

96. (B) Anabolic steroids.

Anabolic steroids are most likely to increase lean body mass. Anabolic steroids mimic the effects of testosterone, a hormone that is naturally produced in the body. One of the effects of testosterone is to promote muscle growth.

97. (B) Overreaching stage.

The General Adaptation Syndrome (GAS) consists of three stages: the alarm stage (initial stress response), the resistance stage (adaptation to stress), and the exhaustion stage (prolonged exposure to stress leading to decreased performance and potential injury).

98. (B) Rectus abdominis.

The muscle commonly referred to as a "six-pack" in athletic individuals is the rectus abdominis. The rectus abdominis is a long, flat muscle that extends vertically along the anterior abdominal wall and is located between the ribs and pubic bone.

99. (A) Plank.

Planks exclusively target the core. Deadlifts and Olympic lifts are exercises that involve multiple muscle groups, including the core, but they are not exclusive to the core. Therefore, the correct answer is option A.

100. (B) Training volume.

Training volume is the measure of the total amount of physical work performed during a workout session or over the course of an exercise program.

101. (C) Construct validity.

Construct validity is often considered the most important and accurate type of validity when evaluating a test. Construct validity refers to the extent to which a test measures the construct or concept it is designed to measure and is typically established through a process of empirical research and analysis.

102. (A) Type I

Type I muscle fibers, also known as slow-twitch fibers, have a high oxidative capacity and are more resistant to fatigue compared to the fast-twitch Type II fibers.

103. (D) The number of repetitions and sets.

In resistance training, "volume" refers to the total number of repetitions and sets performed for a given exercise or muscle group, which is an essential factor in designing training programs to meet specific goals.

104. (A) 18 x 24 inches

The minimum landing surface dimensions for a plyometric box is at least 18 by 24 inches.

105. (B) Optimal functioning theory.

The optimal functioning theory is the theory that explains why some athletes react with excitement and anticipation when experiencing high levels of arousal, rather than with fear and anxiety.

106. (B) Triceps extension.

In a first-class lever, the lever with the fulcrum is located between the effort and resistance. Based on this, the exercise that involves a first-class lever is the triceps extension. In a triceps extension, the elbow joint acts as the fulcrum: the weight being lifted is the resistance, and the effort is provided by the triceps muscles.

107. (D) Synaptic cleft.

The synaptic cleft is a small space between the presynaptic neuron and the postsynaptic cell. It is often referred to as the final component of the NMJ.

108. (C) Increased removal of lactate.

Increased removal of lactate reduces acidic levels in the muscle during intense exercise.

109. (D) Help athletes recover from exercise-induced fatigue and prevent overtraining.

Recovery stages after training help athletes recover from exercise-induced fatigue and prevent overtraining. This allows for better physical and physiological adaptations to endurance training.

110. (C) Strength and power training.

Muscular hypertrophy refers to the increase in size of skeletal muscle fibers through an increase in the size of individual muscle cells. Muscular hypertrophy training is beneficial for strength and power training.

111. (A) By increasing lactate levels.

Alcohol impairs aerobic performance by slowing the citric acid cycle, inhibiting gluconeogenesis, and raising lactate levels. So, option A is correct.

112. (C) Weight loss.

Reported adverse effects of creatine include weight gain due to water retention, muscle strains and pulls, nausea, diarrhea, muscle cramps, muscle stiffness, and heat intolerance. Hence, option C is correct because creatine causes weight gain and not weight loss.

113. (D) The athlete should use a narrower tire.

Offensive and defensive formations tend to be at least 6 ft 1 in. Narrow tires are harder for taller athletes; hence option D is not accurate. The other statements are generally accurate: the tire should be taller than the athlete, the tread surface should be free from exposed metal to avoid injury, and the exercise surface should be hard to provide a stable base for the exercise.

114. (C) Increasing sales of sports equipment.

Increasing sales of sports equipment is not one of the main objectives of sport psychology. Sports psychology is concerned with understanding how psychological factors can influence an athlete's performance. It aims to develop techniques and strategies to help athletes overcome psychological barriers and reach their full potential.

115. (A) Tolerable Upper Intake Level (TUL).

Tolerable Upper Intake Level (TUL) is the maximum daily intake that is unlikely to have a negative impact on health.

116. (B) 16-20 ounces.

It is recommended that athletes drink about 16-20 ounces of water 2 hours before a workout.

117. (D) Severe restriction of food intake.

Severe restriction of food intake is a characteristic of anorexia nervosa. Anorexia nervosa is an eating disorder characterized by a persistent restriction of energy intake, leading to significantly low body weight, an intense fear of gaining weight, and a distorted body image. Compulsive overeating and binge eating followed by purging are characteristics of bulimia nervosa, while craving and eating non-food items is characteristic of pica disorder.

118. (B) Extrinsic motivation.

The correct answer is B. Pursuing a professional sports career for financial gain is a characteristic of extrinsic motivation. Extrinsic motivation refers to motivation that comes from external factors, such as rewards, recognition, or tangible benefits.

119. (C) Calcium and vitamin D.

Calcium and vitamin D are important in optimizing bone density in the elderly population. Calcium is essential for building and maintaining strong bones, while vitamin D helps the body absorb calcium and improve bone health.

120. (C). Allowing the bar to drift away from the body during the lift.

Allowing the bar to drift away from the body during the lift is incorrect. Allowing the bar to drift away from the body can place excessive stress on the lower back and increase the risk of injury.

121. (B) Inhibition of muscle contraction

The Golgi tendon organ is a proprioceptive sensory receptor that senses changes in muscle tension and inhibits muscle contraction to protect against potential injury.

122. (D) Squat.

Closed kinetic chain exercises involve movement with the distal segment of the limb fixed, such as the feet in contact with the ground during a squat. These exercises typically involve multiple joints and muscles working together.

123. (B) Multi-joint exercise.

When starting a resistance training session, it is best to begin with multi-joint exercises, such as squats, deadlifts, and bench presses. These exercises activate multiple muscle groups and require more energy, which helps to activate synergistic muscles, prepare the body for the workout, and increase the production of anabolic hormones.

124. (B) Increased neural drive to muscle fibers.

Increased neural drive to muscle fibers is most likely responsible for the improvement in the athlete's bench press 1 repetition maximum (1RM).

125. (A) Chronological age measures the number of years that have passed, while biological age is a measure of overall growth and development.

126. (D) 2300 milligrams per day.

According to the dietary guidelines for Americans, the daily sodium recommendation is 2300 milligrams per day for adults (that's equal to about 1 teaspoon of table salt). However, the American Heart Association recommends that people with high blood pressure should aim for even lower sodium intakes, around 1500 milligrams per day.

127. (A) Bananas.

Bananas are a good source of potassium, with one medium-sized banana containing approximately 400-450 milligrams of potassium. Pretzels and flax seeds are not significant sources of potassium. In fact, pretzels are relatively high in sodium. White rice is not a significant source of potassium either, especially when compared to other whole grains such as quinoa, brown rice, and barley.

128. (A) Getting regular sun exposure.

Getting regular sun exposure is one of the best ways that athletes can increase their vitamin D levels. Vitamin D is known as the "sunshine vitamin" because the body can produce it when the skin is exposed to sunlight.

129. (D) Hemorrhage.

In adults, athletes taking more than 1,500 IU/day of vitamin E are at an increased risk of hemorrhage.

130. (A) By increasing human growth hormone secretion.

Arginine improves muscle growth by increasing human growth hormone secretion. Reducing inflammation, decreasing blood flow to the muscles, and inhibiting protein synthesis are not ways that arginine improves muscle growth.

131. (B) Beta-hydroxy-beta-methylbutyrate (HMB).

Beta-hydroxy-beta-methylbutyrate (HMB) has been used to promote faster recovery in athletes after exercise. HMB is a metabolite of the amino acid leucine and has been shown to have anti-catabolic effects, which means it can help to reduce muscle breakdown and promote muscle protein synthesis.

132. (C) Enhanced oxygen delivery to muscles.

An important role of iron supplements in exercise is enhanced oxygen delivery to muscles. Iron is a key component of hemoglobin, which is the protein in red blood cells that carries oxygen from the lungs to the muscles.

133. (D) Furosemide.

Diuretics like furosemide have been banned in sports as they are often used as a diuretic and masking agent to hide the use of other performance-enhancing drugs.

134. (A) Hook grip.

The hook grip is the grip recommended for individuals with weak grip strength. The hook grip involves wrapping the thumb around the bar and then wrapping the fingers over the thumb. This creates a secure grip that allows for greater control of the weight and improved grip strength.

135. (A) Increased intra-abdominal pressure.

Increased intra-abdominal pressure is a potential risk associated with the Valsalva maneuver.

136. (C) By increasing the volume of training by adding more sets or reps.

The most effective way to implement progressive overload in a resistance training program is by increasing the volume of training by adding more sets or reps.

137. (A) Low repetition ranges (1-5 reps) are associated with fast-twitch muscle fibers.

Option A is correct because low repetition ranges (1-5 reps) are associated with fast-twitch muscle fibers. Options B, C, and D are inaccurate. Option B is wrong because muscular endurance is typically trained with lighter weights and higher repetitions (15-20+ reps). Option C is inaccurate because there is no such thing as intermediate-twitch muscle fibers. Finally, option D is wrong because low repetition ranges with lighter weights are generally not sufficient for building muscle mass and strength.

138. (B) 3 seconds eccentric, 0 seconds pause, 1 second concentric, 0 seconds pause.

3 seconds eccentric, 0 seconds pause, 1 second concentric, 0 seconds pause is an example of a tempo recommendation. Tempo refers to the speed at which an athlete performs each repetition of an exercise. This recommendation provides specific instructions for the timing of the eccentric (lowering) and concentric (lifting) phases of the exercise, as well as the amount of time to pause between repetitions.

139. (D) The pull.

The "pull" is a key element of the snatch lift. The other movements listed—the press, clean, and jerk—are all separate Olympic weightlifting movements, but are not part of the snatch lift specifically.

140. (C) When the bar is past the knees.

The lifter should accelerate and perform a triple extension of the knees, ankles, and hips when the bar is past the knees during the snatch lift.

141. (A) Requires a significant amount of coaching time and attention.

Olympic lifting requires a significant amount of coaching time and attention due to its technically demanding and complex nature. Exercises such as the snatch and clean and jerk require a great deal of skill and practice to perform correctly and safely.

142. (A) 2.

There are two models of plyometric exercise: the mechanical model and the neurophysiological model.

143. (C) Lower body.

The lower body is the muscle group most commonly targeted in plyometric exercises. Common lower body plyometric exercises include jumping, bounding, and hopping drills, which target the muscles in the legs, hips, and glutes. While upper body and core plyometric exercises do exist, they are less commonly used than lower body plyometric exercises.

144. (D) Muscle endurance.

Muscle endurance is not a key factor in improving speed. The key factors in improving speed are stride frequency and stride length, which determine how quickly an athlete can cover a given distance. The amount of vertical force applied to the ground during the stance phase is considered the most critical component of improving speed.

145. (D) All of the above.

All of the above factors can impact an athlete's recovery needs. Athletes of different ages, genders, and training experiences will have different recovery needs based on their individual physiological and metabolic characteristics.

146. (A) The sport or activity being analyzed.

The first step in a needs analysis is to identify the sport or activity that will be analyzed. Once the sport or activity has been identified, other factors such as the athlete's training history, performance goals, and dietary habits can be evaluated to further inform the design of the training program.

147. (D) All of the above.

The assessment phase of a needs analysis typically involves collecting various types of information about the athlete, including their training history, medical history, and performance goals. This information is used to identify areas where the athlete may need additional training or support and to develop a training plan that is tailored to their specific needs and goals.

148. (C) Analysis of the athlete's cultural background.

The analysis of the athlete's cultural background is not typically included in a sport-specific needs analysis. A sport-specific needs analysis typically includes an assessment of the athlete's current physical condition, an evaluation of the athlete's mental readiness, and an examination of the demands of the sport or activity.

149. (D) By incorporating balance and stability challenges. The progression of unilateral exercises can be modified to increase the training stimulus by incorporating balance and stability challenges.

150. (A) Bench press.

The bench press is not an example of a unilateral exercise. Unilateral exercises are exercises that work one side of the body at a time, and the other three exercises listed—single-arm bicep curls, split squat, and Romanian deadlift—are all examples of unilateral exercises.

151. (C) Isometric.

The method of training that involves holding the muscle in a static position to build strength is called "isometric" training. Isometric training involves contracting a muscle or group of muscles and holding that contraction without any movement of the joints.

152. (C) High-intensity exercise.

When considering the fatigability of the muscles, it is generally recommended to perform high-intensity exercises first in a training session. This is because high-intensity exercises typically require more energy and recruit more muscle fibers and performing them first when the muscles are fresh can help maximize their effectiveness. The correct option is C.

153. (C) Squats.

According to the principle of exercise order, athletes should prioritize compound exercises over isolation exercises, as compound exercises are more demanding and will tire you out faster. Hence, option C is correct. Squats should generally be prioritized first during training because it is a compound exercise that targets multiple muscle groups, including the quadriceps, glutes, and hamstrings.

154. (D) A list of all equipment in the facility.

While it is important to have an inventory of the equipment in the facility for organizational and maintenance purposes, a list of all equipment in the facility is not a key component of the emergency response plan for a strength and conditioning facility.

155. (A) Evacuate the building.

In the event of a fire in a strength and conditioning facility, the first step that should be taken is to evacuate the building immediately. The safety of all individuals in the facility is the top priority.

156. (B) Acceleration.

Acceleration is a key variable to measure in sprint and not agility; hence, it is the correct option. Change-of-direction deficit, ground contact time and exit velocity are all key variables to monitor in agility.

157. (A) Macronutrients are required in larger quantities than micronutrients.

Macronutrients (carbohydrates, fats, and proteins) are required in larger quantities as they provide energy and serve as the building blocks of the body. Micronutrients (vitamins and minerals) are required in smaller quantities and have various roles in maintaining overall health.

158. (C) A verbal warning by a staff member

The first step would be a warning or a verbal warning from a staff member such as the coach, trainer, or any other facility staff member.

159. (C) Verbal abuse by a staff member.

Verbal abuse by a staff member is not a disciplinary measure taken for violating the facility's rules.

160. (D) Medical history.

The first factor among the available options that should be evaluated is the individual's current level of fitness and health, which the individual's medical history provides.

161. (B) Strength phase.

The strength phase of the periodization cycle focuses on developing maximum strength through increased intensity and reduced volume. Exercises during this phase often involve heavy loads and lower repetitions.

162. (C) Third class.

During a push-up exercise, the elbow joint functions as a third-class lever. The fulcrum is the elbow joint, the resistance force is the weight of the body, and the effort force is generated by the contraction of the triceps and other muscles of the arm.

163. (B) Frontal.

During the butterfly stroke in swimming, the abduction of the arms occurs in the frontal plane of action. The arms are moved away from the midline of the body during the pull phase. This movement occurs in the frontal plane, which is the plane that divides the body into front and back halves.

164. (B) 353W.

Power = work ÷ time

Work = force x distance

The force exerted by the weightlifter to lift the barbell is equal to its weight, which is:

Force = mass x gravity

Where mass = 60 kg (the weight of the barbell) and Gravity = 9.81 m/s^2 (the acceleration due to gravity).

Hence, the force exerted by the weightlifter is: force = 60 kg x 9.81 m/s^2 = 588.6 N.

The distance lifted by the weightlifter is 1.5 meters, and they lifted the barbell for 10 repetitions, so the total distance lifted is:

Distance = 1.5 m x 10 = 15 m

Therefore, the work done by the weightlifter is:

Work = force x distance = 588.6 N x 15 m = 8,829 J

Now to calculate the power output:

Power = work ÷ time = 8,829 J ÷ 25 s = 353.16 watts

Therefore, the power output of the weightlifter is 353.16 watts.

So, option B is correct.

165. (A) Biceps brachii

The primary antagonist muscle group during the bench press exercise is the biceps brachii, which is responsible for elbow flexion, opposing the main action of the exercise (elbow extension).

166. (C) Increases the amount of force generated by the quadriceps muscle group.

The patella acts as a fulcrum for the quadriceps muscle group, increasing the lever arm of the knee joint and improving the angle of pull of the quadriceps. This increase allows the quadriceps to produce a greater force at the knee joint with less effort.

167. (A) Lateral raises.

During the lateral raise, the primary movement is abduction of the arms away from the body in the frontal plane.

168. (C) Developing proper technique.

The first priority when incorporating agility drills into the conditioning program of a 15-year-old girl should be developing proper technique. Proper technique is critical when performing agility drills because it helps to reduce the risk of injury and ensures that the exercises are performed correctly and effectively.

169. (D) Resting.

When a muscle is at its resting length or slightly stretched position, there is optimal overlap between the actin and myosin filaments within the muscle fibers. Hence, muscle strength is greatest when the muscle is at its resting length.

170. (A) A muscle unit innervates many muscle fibers.

A motor unit consists of a motor neuron and the muscle fibers it innervates. The number of these muscle fibers can vary from 1 to 1000. Hence, option A is the best option.

171. (D) All of the above.

A dynamic warm-up is designed to increase heart rate, blood flow, flexibility, joint range of motion, and muscle activation, all of which prepare the body for the upcoming workout and reduce the risk of injury.

172. (C) Glutes.

The primary muscle worked in the glute bridge exercise is the gluteus maximus, the largest muscle of the buttocks. The hamstrings might also be worked in the process, but they are secondary. The calves and abs are not directly involved in the glute bridge exercise.

173. (C) A weight bench.

A weight bench or a resistance band is essential for upper body pushing exercises such as bench presses, chest presses, shoulder presses, or triceps presses.

174. (A) Resting on the shoulders.

In the high-bar Olympic squat, the barbell is positioned on the upper traps of the lifter, across the top of the shoulders. So, the correct option is A.

175. (D) Shoulders and the triceps.

The shoulder press exercise, also known as the overhead press, is a compound exercise that primarily targets the deltoid muscles of the shoulders and the triceps muscles of the arms. Hence, option D is correct.

176. (B) Lie on your back with your knees bent and raise your hips toward the ceiling.

The proper form when performing a glute bridge is to lie on your back with your knees bent and raise your hips toward the ceiling.

177. (D). A combination of sport/exercise science, administration, management, teaching, and coaching skills.

Many skills intersecting differently are required in a strength and conditioning professional.

178. (D) The training objectives for the athletes, coaches, and administration.

The training objectives for the athletes, coaches, and administration are the most important aspect of facility design and layout for strength and conditioning coaches.

179. (A) Mental imagery.

The gymnast is engaging in mental imagery, which is the mental rehearsal or visualization of a specific action or movement. This process involves creating a mental image of a specific skill or movement and then mentally rehearsing it in detail, including the sensations, emotions, and feelings associated with it.

180. (B) In linear periodization, training volume and intensity are gradually increased over time, while in undulating periodization, they are alternated on a daily or weekly basis.

The main difference between linear periodization and undulating periodization is how the training volume and intensity are varied over time. In linear periodization, the training volume and intensity are gradually increased over time, often on a weekly or monthly basis. In undulating periodization, the training volume and intensity are alternated on a shorter time scale, typically on a daily or weekly basis.

181. (D) Reverse periodization.

The correct answer is the reverse periodization model. This model begins with a high intensity and low volume and gradually decreases the intensity while increasing the volume over time. It is more commonly used in power and strength sports.

182. (C) A process where risks are explained to participants and they make an informed decision to participate.

Informed consent in sports is a process where the risks and benefits of participation in an activity or event are explained to the participants, and they are given the information they need to make an informed decision about whether or not to participate. Option B looks correct but the concluding statement stated that the participants make an uninformed decision to participate.

183. (A) The phosphagen energy system.

The correct answer is the phosphagen system. The phosphagen energy system is the system that primarily supplies ATP for short, high-intensity activities such as weightlifting or sprinting. This energy system uses stored phosphocreatine to rapidly generate ATP, which can fuel muscle contractions for a short period of time before other energy systems take over.

184. (A) Running a 100-meter dash.

The correct answer is the 100-m dash. The phosphagen energy system would be the primary source of ATP for running a 100-meter dash, which is a short, high-intensity activity that lasts for only a few seconds. For longer-duration activities, such as running a 400-meter dash, running a 1600-meter race, or running a marathon, the phosphagen system would not be sufficient to provide all the needed ATP. The glycolytic and oxidative energy systems are better suited in this case.

185. (B) Depleted muscle glycogen.

Although it is difficult to determine the exact cause of the female gymnast's inability to perform the complicated routine without more information from the available options, depleted muscle glycogen is the most likely factor to limit her performance.

186. (C) Exercise intensity and exercise duration.

Exercise intensity and exercise duration will primarily determine the dominant energy system used during a weightlifting session.

187. (D) The athlete's gender.

The athlete's gender does not affect the recovery time needed for an athlete after a high-intensity interval training session. The duration and intensity of the exercise session are key factors that can affect the amount of stress placed on the body and the amount of time needed for recovery. The athlete's age can also affect recovery time, as older athletes may require longer recovery times due to a decline in muscle mass and reduced ability to recover from high-intensity exercise. So, the best answer is option D.

188. (D) Gastric upset.

At doses greater than 45 mg/day, common side effects of iron include gastric upset, constipation, nausea, abdominal pain, vomiting, and fainting.

189. (B) Marathon running.

Of the options given, marathon running would benefit the most from caffeine supplementation. Endurance sports such as marathon running require prolonged efforts and endurance, making caffeine supplementation a potential benefit for this sport. Caffeine has been shown to improve endurance exercise performance by reducing perceived exertion, increasing alertness and focus, and stimulating the central nervous system.

190. (A) Sphygmomanometer.

The instrument used to measure blood pressure is called a sphygmomanometer.

191. (A). Increased resting heart rate

An increase in resting heart rate is a common indicator of overreaching, which is a state of accumulated fatigue that can lead to a decline in exercise performance.

192. (A) Rapidly swinging the weight to generate momentum.

One of the most commonly made mistakes when performing bicep curls is too much swinging. Hence, the best option A: rapidly swinging the weight to generate momentum. This often occurs when the weight is too heavy or when the individual is trying to perform the exercise too quickly. The problem with this technique is that it shifts the emphasis away from the biceps and places more stress on other muscles and connective tissues, which can increase the risk of injury.

193. (D) All of the above.

All of the options. Understanding organizational trends and best practices in strength and conditioning helps strength and conditioning professionals to stay current with the latest research, implement best practices in their program and provide better training for their athletes.

194. (B) To make sense of data and determine implications for the athlete's training and recovery.

Communicating the results helps to make sense of the data and determine implications for the athlete's training and recovery.

195. (A) To ensure that a test covers the entire range of the construct or variable being measured.

Content validity is used to ensure that a test covers the entire range of the construct or variable being measured.

196. (C) To assess the consistency of test results over time.

Retest involves administering the same test to the same group of people twice and comparing the results. This test is used to assess the consistency of test results over time.

197. (D) High-bar Olympic squat.

The high-bar Olympic squat is a lower body pushing exercise that targets the quadriceps, glutes, and lower back muscles. The bench press is an upper body pushing exercise that primarily targets the chest, triceps, and shoulders, while the shoulder press is another upper body pushing exercise that primarily targets the shoulders and triceps. The deadlift is a lower body pulling exercise that targets the hamstrings, glutes, and lower back muscles. Hence, the correct answer is D.

198. (B) Increase carbohydrate intake, decrease fat, and maintain protein.

To achieve her goal of increasing muscle mass and decreasing body fat, the female bodybuilder should increase carbohydrate intake, decrease fat intake, and maintain protein intake.

199. (C.) T-Test.

The T-Test is the most appropriate test for assessing a male soccer player's agility. This test is specifically designed to assess agility and change-of-direction ability. The 1 RM squat is a test of maximal strength in the lower body, while the 20-meter sprint and standing long jump are measures of speed and power.

200. (A) Leaning too far forward during the descent.

The correct answer is A because leaning too far forward during the descent is a common error while performing the squat. Option B is correct because keeping the feet parallel to each other is a correct technique for the squat, and it helps to maintain proper alignment of the knees and ankles. Fully extending the knees at the top of the movement is also correct, as this represents the top of the movement and helps to complete the repetition. Keeping the feet flat on the ground is also important to maintain proper balance and stability during the exercise.

201. (C) 2-5 minutes.

The recommended rest interval between sets for strength and power training to optimize neuromuscular recovery is 2-5 minutes. Adequate rest intervals are essential for allowing the muscles and nervous system to recover between sets, enabling the athlete to perform at their maximum capacity during subsequent sets.

202. (A) Pull-up.

The pull-up primarily targets the latissimus dorsi muscle, which is responsible for shoulder extension, adduction, and internal rotation. This large back muscle is essential for many pulling movements.

203. (A) I only.

The correct answer is I only. Push-ups primarily target the chest muscles, while bicep curls primarily target the bicep muscles. Lunges and squats primarily target the lower body muscles.

204. (C). I, II, and IV only.

The correct answer is option C: I, II, and IV only. High-intensity interval training (HIIT) involves short, intense bursts of exercise followed by periods of rest or active recovery. This type of training has been shown to improve cardiovascular fitness, as it increases the heart rate and challenges the cardiovascular system. HIIT also burns more calories than steady-state cardio, as it elevates the metabolic rate for hours after the workout.

205. (C) Jumps in place → box jumps → depth jumps

For a beginner, it is most appropriate to progress plyometric exercises from lower-intensity exercises to higher-intensity exercises. A suggested progression would be starting with jumps in place, then moving to box jumps, and finally progressing to depth jumps.

206. (B) To stabilize the shoulder joint

The main function of the rotator cuff muscles is to stabilize the shoulder joint (option B). The rotator cuff is a group of four muscles—supraspinatus, infraspinatus, teres minor, and subscapularis—that originate from the scapula (shoulder blade) and attach to the humerus (upper arm bone). These muscles work together to keep the head of the humerus firmly within the shallow glenoid cavity of the scapula, providing stability to the shoulder joint during various arm movements.

207. (D). Pause and work on improving hip and ankle mobility before attempting the next repetition. It is advised that the athlete pause and work on improving hip and ankle mobility before attempting the next repetition.

208. (B) Stabilization of the spine.

The primary function of the abdominal muscles during a squat is to stabilize the spine by maintaining a neutral position and preventing excessive flexion, extension, or lateral flexion.

209. (A) The time between sets of an exercise.

The rest interval refers to the time between sets of an exercise. Rest intervals allow for recovery between sets and can be adjusted depending on the training goals, intensity, and volume of the workout.

210. (B) Neutral grip with palms facing each other.

The recommended hand position for a barbell overhead press is a neutral grip with palms facing each other. This grip helps to ensure proper alignment of the wrists, elbows, and shoulders, which allows for optimal force production and reduces the risk of injury.

211. (C) Autogenic training involves replacing the muscle relaxation cycle with a focus on feelings of warmth and heaviness, while progressive muscle relaxation involves alternating tensing and relaxing different muscle groups.

Autogenic training involves replacing the muscle relaxation cycle with a focus on feelings of warmth and heaviness, while progressive muscle relaxation involves alternating tensing and relaxing different muscle groups.

212. (B) Holding your breath and bearing down to increase intra-abdominal pressure during heavy lifting.

The Valsalva maneuver is a technique used during weightlifting, where the lifter takes a deep breath, holds it, and bears down (by contracting the muscles of the abdomen) to create increased intra-abdominal pressure. Hence, the correct answer is B.

213. (B) 195.

The estimated maximum age-predicted heart rate would be calculated as 220 − age (years)= beats per minute (bpm).

So, for a 25-year-old:

Maximum heart rate = 220 - 25 = 195 beats per minute.

214. (C) The knee cap (patella).

The knee cap (patella) is the part of the body that enhances the performance of the quadriceps muscle group. It does this by keeping the tendon away from the center of rotation at the knee. In summary, the patella acts as a fulcrum, allowing the quadriceps muscle to generate more force during knee extension movements.

215. (B) Standing upright with arms at the sides and facing forward.

The anatomical position of the human body is standing upright with arms at the sides and facing forward. The feet are shoulder-width apart, and the body is standing straight with the head and eyes looking straight ahead. This position is commonly used as a reference point for describing the location and orientation of various structures within the body.

216. (B) The jerk.

The final portion of the clean and jerk lift is called the jerk. During the jerk, the lifter takes the weight from the front rack position (where the bar is resting on the shoulders) and uses a quick dip and drive with the legs to generate momentum, followed by a strong press with the arms to complete the lift.

217. (C) Increased capillary density.

Increased capillary density can delay muscle fatigue by providing more efficient oxygen delivery and removal of waste products from working muscles. Decreased stroke volume, and decreased hemoglobin levels, can both contribute to reduced oxygen delivery to the muscles and increase the risk of muscle fatigue. Increased oxygen uptake can also help delay muscle fatigue by improving the efficiency of oxygen delivery to the muscles. However, it does this to a lesser extent than increased capillary density, so option C is the best answer.

218. (C) Increased mitochondrial density.

Training increases the number and size of mitochondria within slow-twitch muscle fibers, which improves their oxidative capacity and enhances their ability to produce energy aerobically. Additionally, it's worth noting that options A, B, and D are adaptations more commonly associated with fast-twitch muscle fibers rather than slow-twitch muscle fibers.

219. (B) 225 pounds.

The appropriate training load for the client if the program calls for 75% of their one-rep max (300 pounds) would be 225 pounds.

To calculate the appropriate training load, we can use the formula:

Training load = One-rep max x % of one-rep max

Training load = 300 pounds x 0.75 = 225 pounds

Therefore, the appropriate training load for the client in this case would be 225 pounds. Hence option C is correct.

220. (B) 110 pounds.

Estimated one-rep max = weight lifted / (1.0278 - 0.0278 x number of repetitions)

Estimated one-rep max = 80 pounds / (1.0278 - 0.0278 x 8) = 110 pounds

Therefore, based on the Brzycki formula, the estimated one-rep max for the client would be approximately 110 pounds.

Hence, the correct answer is B.

Test 2 Questions

1. Which of the following muscles is responsible for chewing?

A. Orbicularis oris

B. Buccinator

C. Temporalis

D. Platysma

2. Joints found in sutures of the skull are examples of what type of joints?

A. Fibrous joint

B. Synovial joint

C. Cartilaginous joints

D. Regular joints

3. Which of the following substances must be present for myosin and actin cross bridges to function properly?

A. Manganese and fructose

B. Calcium and ATP

C. Calcium and sucrose

D. ATP and sucrose

4. Which of the following neurons are responsible for sending electrical signals from the brain to the muscles?

A. Motor neurons

B. Sensory neurons

C. Interneurons

D. Intraneurons

5. What is the role of the perisynaptic Schwann cells in the Neuromuscular Junction?

A. They participate in muscle contraction

B. They help neurons communicate with other cells

C. They help in the development, maintenance, and repair of the synapse

D. They break down acetylcholine

6. Which of these biomechanical principles measures how difficult it is to change an object's state of motion?

A. The principle of range of motion

B. The principle of inertia

C. The principle of balance

D. The principle of coordination continuum

7. What type of muscle makes up the majority of the total body weight in humans?

A. Cardiac muscle

B. Smooth muscle

C. Skeletal muscle

D. All of the above

8. Which of the following is true about the phosphagen energy system?

A. This system uses carbohydrates or fat to generate ATP

B. It is anaerobic or oxygen-independent

C. It is not sufficient short-term, intense activities

D. It is great for endurance exercises

9. Which of these organs prevents aspiration?

A. Epiglottis

B. Pharynx

C. Alveoli

D. Trachea

10. Which of the following is the most abundant type of connective tissue in the body?

A. Osseous tissue

B. Loose connective tissue

C. Dense connective tissue

D. Adipose connective tissue

11. The portion of the blood that is pumped out of the heart with each contraction is referred to as_____.

A. Stroke volume

B. Ejection fraction

C. Diastolic volume

D. Systolic volume

12. Which of the following types of stretching is most appropriate to perform during a cool-down after a workout?

A. Ballistic stretching

B. Dynamic stretching

C. Static stretching

D. PNF stretching

13. Which of these is also referred to as the pacemaker of the heart?

A. The AV node

B. The Purkinje fibers

C. The SA node

D. The Bundle of His

14. Which of the following energy systems produces ATP at the fastest rate?

A. Phosphagen

B. Fat oxidation

C. Aerobic glycolysis

D. Anaerobic glycolysis

15. Which of the following activities would be considered low impact?

A. Running

B. Cycling

C. Jumping jacks

D. Plyometric exercises

16. Which principle of biomechanics refers to the ability to control body position in relation to the base of support?

A. The principle of coordination continuum

B. The principle of optimal projection

C. The principle of balance

D. The principle of segmental interaction

17. What is the principle of force-motion in biomechanics based on?

A. Leibniz theory

B. Newton's first law of motion

C. Bernoulli's principle

D. Archimedes' principle

18. How many bones are found in the human skeleton?

A. 126

B. 206

C. 80

D. 216

19. The influx of what substance causes the myosin heads to crosslink with the actin so that muscle contraction can begin?

A. Sodium influx

B. Calcium influx

C. Magnesium influx

D. Potassium influx

20. All these are muscles found in the upper extremity, except?

A. Trapezius

B. Brachioradialis

C. Subclavius muscle

D. Pyramidalis

21. All these are examples of isotonic exercises except?

A. Cycling

B. Weight lifting

C. Swimming

D. Running

22. Which of the following is the main site of neuroendocrine interaction in the human body?

A. The liver

B. The pancreas

C. The hypothalamus and pituitary

D. The adrenal glands

23. Athletes who consume excessive alcohol are likely to be deficient in which of these vitamins?

A. Vitamin D

B. Vitamin B1

C. Vitamin E

D. Vitamin A

24. Which of these is the recommended dietary allowance (RDA) of magnesium for a 21-year female basketballer?

A. 400-420mg

B. 3500-4700mg

C. 310-320 mg

D. 4000-4290 mg

25. Which of the following motivations is driven by an athlete's desire to participate in a competition and compare their performance with others?

A. Intrinsic motivation

B. Extrinsic motivation

C. Achievement motivation

D. Incentivized motivation

26. The bones in the vertebrae and skull are _____ bones.

A. Short bones

B. Long bones

C. Flat bones

D. Irregular bones

27. Which exercises primarily target the biceps?

A. Tricep extensions

B. Hammer curls

C. Lat pulldowns

D. Deadlifts

28. Which of the following muscles is an antagonist during a biceps curl?

A. Brachioradialis muscle

B. Triceps

C. Deltoids

D. Pectoralis

29. What is the primary way that beta-alanine improves exercise performance?

A. By increasing muscle strength

B. By reducing muscle fatigue

C. By improving oxygen delivery to muscles

D. By increasing energy production in muscles

30. Which anatomical plane separates the left and right halves of the body?

A. Sagittal plane

B. Cross-plane

C. Horizontal plane

D. Forefront plane

31. During a 400m run, which of the following is the most probable limiting factor?

A. Liver glycogen

B. Fat stores

C. Creatine phosphate

D. Muscle glycogens

32. Which of the following accurately defines the eating disorder called pica?

A. The persistent eating of non-nutritive, non-food substances for at least a month.

B. The persistent eating of only one type of food for at least a month

C. The persistent eating of an excessive amount of food for at least a month

D. The persistent eating of only vegetables and fruits for at least a month

33. Which of the following is the mathematical representation of stroke volume?

A. SV = EDV + ESV

B. SV = EDV−ESV

C. SV = EDV × ESV

D. SV = EDV/ ESV

34. Which of the following nutrients is most important for an athlete's recovery and tissue repair?

A. Carbohydrates

B. Proteins

C. Vitamin B1

D. Fats

35. The basic functional unit of the nervous system is referred to as_____.

A. Nephrons

B. Neurons

C. Axons

D. Dendrons

36. Which of these is a neural strategy for promoting recovery in an athlete?

A. Hydration

B. Massage

C. Cryotherapy

D. Use of compression garments

37. Which of the following is Cunningham's equation for calculating Resting Metabolic Rate (RMR)?

A. RMR = Body Weight x 15 + 6.25 x Height (cm)

B. RMR = Body Weight x 10 + 22 x free fat mass(kg)

C. RMR = Body Mass x 9.99 + 6.25 x Height (cm) - 4.92 x Age (years) + 5

D. RMR = 500 + 22 x free fat mass(kg)

38. The practice of eliminating a previously established consequence for an athlete's behavior following a successful performance is referred to as:

A. Positive reinforcement

B. Negative reinforcement

C. Achievement motivation

D. Intrinsic motivation

39. All of these athletes except one have more type I fibers in their muscle cells.

A. Cross-country runners

B. Weight lifters

C. Endurance swimmers

D. Long-distance cyclers

40. Which of the following substances plays an important role in muscle contraction?

A. Potassium

B. Magnesium

C. Phosphorus

D. Calcium

41. Which of the following is not a characteristic of muscle cells?

A. Excitability

B. Elasticity

C. Reflexibility

D. Contractility

42. When a molecule of glucose is broken down into pyruvate using glycolysis, _____ molecules of ATP are produced in the process.

A. 36

B. 2

C. 38

D. 4

43. _____ is the chief neurotransmitter in the parasympathetic nervous system.

A. Epinephrine

B. Catecholamine

C. Norepinephrine

D. Acetylcholine

44. In which body position is the rectus abdominis muscle most effectively activated during a crunch exercise?

A. Legs flat on the ground

B. Legs bent at 90 degrees with feet on the ground

C. Legs bent at 90 degrees with feet elevated

D. Legs straight up in the air

45. Which pathway provides the greatest supply of ATP in the final phase of a marathon race?

A. Aerobic respiration

B. Oxidation of fats

C. Phosphocreatine system

D. Glycolysis

46. Which of these periodization cycles is a medium-length cycle, typically lasting several weeks to a few months?

A. Macrocycle

B. Microcycle

C. Epicycle

D. Mesocycle

47. Which of the following best describes a supinated grip in resistance training?

A. Palms upward when grasping the bar

B. Middle and index fingers grasping the bar

C. Palms are facing down

D. All of the above

48. What type of lever is seen during a bicep curl?

A. Third class lever

B. Fourth class lever

C. First class lever

D. All of the above

49. Which of these white blood cells take part in allergic inflammatory reactions?

A. Lymphocytes

B. Monocytes

C. Eosinophils

D. Neutrophils

50. Push-ups, pull-ups, and chin-ups are examples of what type of exercise?

A. Bodyweight

B. Core stability

C. Flexibility

D. Balance

51. Which of the following is not one of the main techniques for tire flipping?

A. The sumo

B. Backlift style

C. The log-lift

D. Shoulders-against-the-tire technique

52. Which of the following forms of exercise involves doing a sequence of exercises back-to-back without rest, repeated multiple times?

A. Progressive overload

B. High-intensity training

C. Circuit training

D. Isometric training

53. Which of the following relaxation techniques involves the repetition of phrases and visualization to bring about a state of deep relaxation?

A. Progressive Muscle Relaxation (PMR)

B. Autogenic training

C. Deep breathing exercise

D. Guided imagery

54. Which of the following provides an analysis of the sport's injury risks, which helps the coach to design training programs that can help prevent such injuries?

A. Exercise selection

B. Mechanical analysis

C. NEEDs analysis

D. Strength evaluation

55. What type of exercise is the barbell biceps curl classified as?

A. Assistance exercise

B. Core exercise

C. Plyometric exercise

D. Multi-joint exercise

56. You are setting up a series of plyometric drills for the men's baseball team; which of the following surfaces is best suited for this type of training?

A. Hardwood surfaces

B. Thick exercise mats

C. Tiles

D. Suspended wood floor

57. Which of the following defines the relationship between force and time?

A. Velocity

B. Acceleration

C. Impulse

D. Momentum

58. Short rest periods are recommended for all of these exercises except?

A. Powerlifting

B. Weight lifting

C. Plyometrics

D. Sprints

59. When designing a strength and conditioning facility, mirrors should be positioned at least how many inches away from equipment?

A. 6

B. 12

C. 20

D. 22

60. An athlete performing 3 to 4 sets of 8-10 repetitions of the same exercise is most likely trying to increase which of the following?

A. Muscle power

B. Muscle hypertrophy

C. Muscle strength

D. Muscle endurance

61. Which of the following floors are not recommended for plyometric exercises?

A. Grass fields

B. Concrete

C. Suspended floors

D. Rubber mats

62. _____ is defined as the relationship between mass and velocity.

A. Speed

B. Force

C. Impulse

D. Momentum

63. What is the primary purpose of incorporating a tapering period before a competition?

A. To increase the training volume

B. To reduce the risk of overtraining

C. To promote peak performance

D. To focus on skill development

64. In which phase of the General Adaptation Syndrome (GAS) does the body adapt to the training stimulus and return to a state of equilibrium?

A. Alarm phase

B. Resistance phase

C. Exhaustion phase

D. Recovery phase

65. During which sports season should a coach focus on improving weaknesses and maintaining the strengths of the athlete?

A. Post-season

B. Pre-season

C. Off-season

D. In-season

66. What energy system is utilized majorly in endurance cycling?

A. Glycolytic system

B. Phosphagen system

C. Oxidative system

D. Concentric system

67. Which of these temperature ranges is ideal for a strength and conditioning facility?

A. 64-68°F

B. 68-78°F

C. 78-82°F

D. 78-84°F

68. Which of these performance-enhancing substances is used as a masking agent to avoid detection of another banned substance?

A. Erythropoietin

B. Ephedrine

C. Diuretics

D. Creatine

69. How should an athlete's macronutrient intake be adjusted during a period of reduced training volume or tapering?

A. Increase carbohydrate intake

B. Decrease carbohydrate intake

C. Maintain consistent macronutrient intake

D. Increase protein intake

70. In the context of strength training, what is meant by "training age"?

A. The number of years a person has been consistently training in a structured and supervised program

B. The amount of time a person has been actively participating in weightlifting competitions

C. The amount of time a person has been consistently practicing weightlifting without formal instruction or supervision

D. The number of weightlifting sessions a person has completed in their lifetime

71. Which body part is not considered one of the five points of contact during seated or supine exercises on a bench?

A. Buttocks

B. Head

C. Left foot

D. Lower back

72. What is the correct form for a deadlift exercise?

A. Hips lower than knees, back rounded, toes pointing forward

B. Hips higher than knees, back straight, toes pointing forward

C. Hips lower than knees, back straight, toes pointing to the sides

D. Hips higher than knees, back rounded, toes pointing to the sides

73. All of these are factors that can contribute to mental health issues in athletes, except?

A. Genetic predisposition to mental health issues

B. Injuries or chronic pain

C. Performance anxiety

D. None of the above

74. Athletes who avoid dairy may struggle to meet which of the following dietary requirements?

A. Fiber

B. Carbohydrates

C. Calcium

D. Vitamin C

75. Which of the following is a characteristic of bulimia nervosa?

A. Binge eating followed by purging

B. Refusal to eat

C. Overeating without purging

D. Craving and eating non-food items

76. Which exercise is typically considered to be the best choice to perform first in a resistance training session?

A. Bench press

B. Power clean

C. Deadlift

D. Lat pulldown

77. A 17-year-old athlete who has been working with a strength and conditioning coach for 3 years has expressed interest in using creatine. The coach is asked for advice on which brand to use. What is the appropriate response?

A. Advise against the use of creatine

B. Suggest any well-known brand

C. Recommend that the athlete seeks advice from a knowledgeable nutritionist or dietitian

D. Suggest the athlete try the brand of creatine the coach uses personally

78. A weightlifter wants to increase her muscle mass and strength. Currently, her daily caloric intake of 2,800 has allowed her to maintain a body weight of 60 kg. In order to gain 4 kg of lean body mass, she should adhere to which of the following guidelines each day?

A. Consume 250 additional kilocalories and 96 g of protein

B. Consume 400 additional kilocalories and 128 g of protein

C. Consume 250 additional kilocalories and 72 g of protein

D. Consume 400 additional kilocalories and 80 g of protein

79. Which of the following is a banned substance that is commonly used to increase alertness and reduce fatigue?

A. Creatine

B. Caffeine

C. Furosemide

D. Nitric oxide

80. Which of the following is a hormone that is naturally produced by the body and is often used to treat certain medical conditions but is also abused by athletes to increase muscle mass and strength?

A. Insulin

B. Thyroid hormone

C. Cortisol

D. Growth hormone

81. What is the function of the Valsalva maneuver during weightlifting exercises?

A. To increase blood flow to the working muscles

B. To reduce the risk of injury

C. To improve breathing efficiency

D. To provide a stable foundation for lifting heavy loads

82. Which of the following is a potential drawback of using progressive overload in a resistance training program?

A. Increased risk of injury if load or exercise is done too frequently

B. Decreased motivation and adherence to the program

C. Stagnation in strength and muscle gains due to overtraining

D. None of the above

83. In strength training, _____ refers to the speed at which an exercise is performed.

A. Reps

B. Sets

C. Tempo

D. Velocity

84. Which of these represents the eccentric phase:

A. The portion of the exercise where the muscle shortens

B. The portion of the exercise where the muscle lengthens

C. The portion of the exercise where the muscle contracts

D. The portion of the exercise where the muscle relaxes

85. How does the patella enhance the performance of the quadriceps muscle group?

A. By decreasing the length of the moment arm

B. By keeping the tendon away from the center of rotation at the knee

C. By increasing the resistance during flexion

D. By transferring energy across body segments

86. A 40-year-old male athlete is aerobically exercising at 80-90% of his functional capacity. The heart rate at rest is 68 bpm. Calculate the target heart rate range according to the Karvonen method.

A. 158-169 bpm

B. 170-185 bpm

C. 190-205 bpm

D. 210-225 bpm

87. Which of the following is an example of a plyometric exercise?

A. Bicep curl

B. Lat pulldown

C. Box drills

D. Tricep extension

88. How should you grip the barbell when performing a sumo deadlift?

A. With a narrow, overhand grip

B. With a wide, overhand grip

C. With a mixed grip

D. With a narrow, underhand grip

89. What type of training is used to develop the ability to change direction quickly?

A. Agility training

B. Plyometric training

C. Speed training

D. Strength training

90. What is the primary purpose of a needs analysis in sports training?

A. To evaluate the athlete's disabilities

B. To identify areas where the athlete needs improvement

C. To assess the athlete's psychological readiness for training

D. To establish the athlete's dietary requirements

91. Which of the following is not typically included in a needs analysis for athlete-specific training?

A. Movement assessment

B. Injury history

C. Dietary preferences

D. Exercise history

92. What is the recommended exercise order when performing a resistance training workout?

A. Compound exercises before isolation exercises

B. Upper body exercises before lower body exercises

C. Lighter weight exercises before heavier weight exercises

D. Static stretches before dynamic stretches

93. Which of these is not a type of speed drill?

A. A-skip

B. Z-drill

C. Fast feet

D. Sprint resistance

94. What of the following is the penalty for a third offense of violating the facility's rules?

A. Dismissal from the facility for one day

B. Dismissal from the facility for one week

C. Dismissal from the facility for the remainder of the year

D. Permanent dismissal from the facility

95. Which of the following exercises is primarily used to strengthen the transverse plane?

A. Bicep curls

B. Lunges

C. Russian twists

D. Shoulder press

96. An athlete is performing a clean and jerk with a weight of 100 kg. If the athlete completes the lift in 4 seconds, what is their power output?

A. 490 W

B. 1000 W

C. 1,500 W

D. 2,000 W

97. Which of the following hormones is primarily responsible for stimulating muscle protein synthesis?

A. Cortisol

B. Insulin

C. Testosterone

D. Growth hormone

98. Which of the following exercises primarily targets the quadriceps muscle group?

A. Leg curl

B. Leg extension

C. Deadlift

D. Glute bridge

99. When performing a barbell bench press, which of the following grip types is recommended for optimal performance?

A. Narrow, underhand grip

B. Wide, overhand grip

C. Narrow, overhand grip

D. Mixed grip

100. What is the primary factor that determines an athlete's ability to generate force in executing movement techniques?

A. Mass

B. Velocity

C. Acceleration

D. Rate of force development

101. Which of the following best describes the concept of super-compensation in relation to exercise training?

A. Supercompensation is a process by which muscle fibers are broken down during exercise and rebuilt stronger during recovery

B. Supercompensation is the temporary decrease in performance that occurs immediately following a period of high-intensity exercise

C. Supercompensation is a process by which the body overcompensates for the stress of exercise, resulting in increased levels of strength and endurance

D. Supercompensation is a process by which the body adapts to a specific exercise stimulus, becoming more resistant to future stress

102. What is the proper grip for the barbell when performing a high-bar Olympic squat?

A. Narrow, underhand grip

B. Wide, overhand grip

C. Narrow, overhand grip

D. Wide, underhand grip

103. What can understanding organizational trends and best practices in strength and conditioning help a strength and conditioning specialist do?

A. Stay current with the latest research

B. Implement best practices in their program

C. Provide better training for their athletes

D. All of the above

104. What is the purpose of incorporating sport seasons into the periodization cycles?

A. To organize the daily and weekly training schedule

B. To focus on specific training goals and objectives

C. To plan and organize the overall training program

D. To adapt the training program to the specific demands of the sport and optimize performance

105. Which of these statements defines the term "assumption of risk" in sports?

A. Acknowledgement of inherent risk in participating and choosing not to participate

B. Acknowledgement of inherent risk in participating and choosing to participate anyway

C. Acknowledgement of no risk in participating and choosing to participate

D. Acknowledgement of no risk in participating and choosing not to participate

106. What is the primary function of creatine supplementation in strength and conditioning?

A. Increase muscle protein synthesis

B. Enhance aerobic capacity

C. Reduce muscle soreness

D. Improve short-term, high-intensity performance

107. A 40-year-old runner is doing a tempo run. Which of the following does not affect his heart rate?

A. The duration of his exercise session

B. Male gender

C. His state of training

D. His initial caffeine levels

108. What is the primary goal of a dynamic warm-up?

A. To increase muscle temperature and blood flow

B. To improve flexibility through static stretching

C. To activate the central nervous system

D. Both A and C

109. Which of the following is NOT a factor that affects an individual's flexibility?

A. Muscle temperature

B. Joint structure

C. Age

D. Hydration status

110. Which of the following are benefits of resistance training?

I. Increases muscle mass and strength

II. Helps maintain bone density

III. Improves joint flexibility

IV. Can be performed at home without equipment

A. I and II

B. II and III

C. I, II, and IV

D. I, III, and IV

111. A bodybuilder would like to train a 10RM load in the dumbbell curl with the addition of a resistance band. Presently, the athlete's 10RM is 45 lbs. How much weight should be used if the athlete applies a 20 lb. resistance band?

A. 25 lbs.

B. 35 lbs.

C. 40 lbs.

D. 50 lbs.

112. What are the variables used in Cunningham's equation to calculate RMR?

A. Body weight and height (cm)

B. Body weight and free fat mass (kg)

C. Body mass, age (years), and free fat mass (kg)

D. None of the above

113. Which of the following physiological adaptations leads to an increase in the amount of oxygen transported into the blood for the muscle's use during aerobic activity?

A. Increased stroke volume

B. Increased oxygen uptake

C. Increased hemoglobin levels

D. Increased capillary density

114. A 25-year-old weightlifter is performing a strength training workout, which of the following does not affect his muscle fatigue?

A. The number of sets he performs

B. His gender

C. His state of training

D. His initial hydration levels

115. What type of reliability test is used to measure the consistency of scores across raters or test forms?

A. Test-retest reliability

B. Alternate-form reliability

C. Split-half reliability

D. Intra-rater reliability

116. _____ characteristics of muscle depict their ability to react to stimulus.

A. Contractility

B. Extensibility

C. Excitability

D. Elasticity

117. The skeletal muscle is attached to the bones through_____?

A. Joint

B. Tendon

C. Ligament

D. None of the following

118. All these are muscles found in the upper extremities, except?

A. Biceps brachii

B. Triceps brachii

C. Deltoid

D. Quadratus femoris

119. All of the following include the muscles that make up the glutes, except?

A. Gluteus maximus

B. Gluteus ilium

C. Gluteus minimus

D. Gluteus medius

120. Splinters have an abundance of _____ fibers?

A. Type I

B. Type IIA

C. Type IIB

D. None of the options

121. Cartilaginous joints are composed solely of _____ cartilage.

A. Collage

B. Hyaline

C. Elastic

D. Membranous

122. Which of these is a way the skeletal muscle adapts to mechanical overload?

A. Decreased mitochondrial density

B. Increased protein synthesis

C. Increased muscle fiber atrophy

D. Decreased myofibrillar hypertrophy

123. Which of these will endurance training most likely target?

A. Increase muscle size

B. Improved myofibrillar protein synthesis

C. Improved aerobic metabolism

D. Decreased mitochondrial density

124. All of the following are characteristics of short bones, except?

A. Thin

B. Flattened

C. Cube shaped

D. Slightly curved

125. Which of these statements is false about brown connective tissue?

A. It appears as a large unilocular lipid droplet under a microscope

B. It generates heat by consuming energy reserves in the body

C. It is often found in infants

D. It decreases with age

126. Which of these connective tissue lacks fibers?

A. Cartilage

B. Blood

C. Elastic tissue

D. Loose tissue

127. Which of these statements is correct when the mechanical advantage is greater than 1?

A. The resistive force is less than the applied force

B. The resistive force is greater than the applied force

C. The resistive force is equal to the applied force

D. None of the following

128. Which of the following statements is true regarding body size and muscle strength?

A. Larger individuals will always be stronger than smaller individuals

B. Body size has no impact on muscle strength

C. Smaller individuals may have an advantage in strength-to-weight ratio

D. Muscle strength is determined solely by genetics and is not impacted by body size

129. Which of the following training modalities is most effective for increasing muscle size and strength?

A. Low-intensity, high-volume endurance training

B. High-intensity, low-volume strength training

C. High-intensity, high-volume powerlifting-style training

D. Yoga and other flexibility-focused exercise

130. Overhead lifts pose the greatest risk to which of these body parts?

A. Knees

B. Elbows and wrists

C. Shoulders

D. Ankles

131. All of these are steps to take to reduce risk of injury in athletes, except?

A. Warm up with heavy weights

B. Avoid maximal loads without proper preparation

C. Incorporate variation and be mindful of pain

D. Be careful when adding plyometric drills to the training program

132. _____ refers to the total sum of all chemical reactions in a biological system.

A. Anabolism

B. Metabolism

C. Catabolism

D. Anachronism

133. Which of the following workout techniques works out a specific body area by interspersing predetermined periods of exercise and rest?

A. Circuit training

B. Plyometric training

C. Interval training

D. Resistance training

134. Which of the following muscles is primarily responsible for inhalation during normal breathing?

A. Diaphragm

B. External intercostals

C. Internal intercostals

D. Rectus abdominis

135. Which of the following structures is responsible for filtering and warming incoming air?

A. Alveoli

B. Bronchioles

C. Nasal cavity

D. Trachea

136. Blood is made up of how many percent of plasma?

A. 25%

B. 35%

C. 45%

D. 55%

137. Which of the following is not a component of the cardiovascular system?

A. Heart

B. Lungs

C. Blood vessels

D. Spleen

138. What is the name of the muscular layer of the heart?

A. Endocardium

B. Pericardium

C. Myocardium

D. Epicardium

139. _____ receives oxygenated blood from the lungs and drains it into the left atrium.

A. Superior vena cava

B. Inferior vena cava

C. Pulmonary artery

D. Pulmonary vein

140. Which of the following structures is not a part of the cardiac conduction system?

A. Sinoatrial (SA) node

B. Atrioventricular (AV) node

C. Atria

D. Ventricles

141. What is the correct sequence of the movement of the electrical impulse generated by the sinoatrial (SA) node?

A. Atria first, then the ventricles

B. Ventricles first, then the atria

C. Both the atria and ventricles simultaneously

D. None of the above

142. The period of time during the cardiac cycle when the heart is relaxed and filling with blood is called:

A. Systole

B. Diastole

C. Ejection phase

D. Preload

143. Which of the following figures depicts high blood pressure?

A. 90/60mmHg

B. 120/80mmHg

C. 130/90mmHg

D. 140/90mmHg

144. What is the primary function of the triceps brachii muscle?

A. Flexion of the elbow joint

B. Extension of the elbow joint

C. Adduction of the arm at the shoulder joint

D. Rotation of the forearm

145. Which of the following is a benefit of incorporating balance and stability exercises into a strength and conditioning program?

A. Improved muscular endurance

B. Enhanced proprioception and neuromuscular control

C. Increased muscle mass

D. Faster recovery between workouts

146. Which of the following is one of the physiological adaptations that helps decrease the resting heart rate in athletes?

A. Decreased stroke volume

B. Increased stroke volume

C. Decreased oxygen capacity

D. Increased oxygen capacity

147. Increased stroke volume directly results in which of the following?

A. Increased cardiac output

B. Increased oxygen capacity

C. Increased protein synthesis

D. Increased lactate threshold

148. Which of the following is one of the major reasons why oxygen uptake increases during exercise/training?

I. Increase in hemoglobin

II. Increase myoglobin levels.

III. Increased protein synthesis

A. I only

B. I and II

C. II and III

D. I, II, and III

149. Which of the following people have the greatest adaptation potential and show rapid gains in strength or endurance?

A. People who have trained for three-five years

B. People who have just started training

C. People who have trained for more than 10 years

D. People who have no prior training experience

150. Which of the following is an effective recovery method for reducing delayed onset muscle soreness?

A. Active recovery

B. Cryotherapy

C. Compression garments

D. All of the above

151. Which of the following is the most effective way to increase power in athletes?

A. Increasing muscular endurance

B. Focusing on high repetition sets with low weights

C. Incorporating plyometric exercises

D. Performing static stretching before workouts

152. Which of the following is a recommended approach for promoting recovery after resistance training?

A. Performing high-intensity interval training (HIIT)

B. Incorporating long-duration, low-intensity cardio

C. Varying the type and intensity of exercises

D. Using low weight, high repetition sets

153. Which of the following is an effective recovery method for promoting muscle repair and reducing inflammation?

A. Active recovery

B. Cryotherapy

C. Static stretching

D. Debriefing

154. All these are important requirements in patients with disability, except?

A. Modified facilities

B. Adapted equipment

C. Personal assistants or interpreters

D. All of the options are important

155. Which of the following is a key component of achievement motivation?

A. Perceived competence

B. Anxiety

C. Social support

D. Internal locus of control

156. What are some common psychological symptoms that may indicate a mental health issue in athletes?

A. Poor coordination and balance

B. Reduced performance

C. Feelings of sadness or anxiety

D. Increased heart rate and blood pressure

157. Which of the following is a potential risk factor for mental health issues in athletes?

A. High levels of social support

B. Low levels of perfectionism

C. Chronic pain or injury

D. Consistent success in competition

158. Which of the following macronutrients provides the highest amount of energy per gram?

A. Protein

B. Carbohydrates

C. Fats

D. Fiber

159. Which of the following micronutrients is important for bone health and can be found in dairy products, leafy greens, and fortified foods?

A. Vitamin D

B. Iron

C. Zinc

D. Magnesium

160. Which of the following is a healthy source of dietary fat?

A. Fructose

B. Sucrose

C. Monounsaturated fats

D. All of the above

161. _____ is an eating disorder in which an individual craves and eats non-food items, such as paper, chalk, or dirt.

A. Rumination disorder

B. Pica

C. Bulimia

D. Anorexia

162. 1g of alcohol equals _____ Kcals of energy.

A. 4

B. 5

C. 7

D. 9

163. How many calories will a protein bar have if the protein bar has the following macros: protein: 40 grams, carbs: 10 grams and fat: 2.5 grams?

A. 223 calories

B. 303 calories

C. 404 calories

D. 504 calories

164. What is the recommended timing for fluid consumption during exercise to prevent dehydration?

A. Before exercise

B. During exercise

C. After exercise

D. Before and after exercise only

165. Beta-alanine is commonly used as a supplement to enhance:

A. Muscle strength

B. Endurance performance

C. Recovery time

D. Cognitive function

166. Which of the following is a common side effect of anabolic steroid use in women?

A. Deepening of the voice

B. Decreased breast size

C. Increased body hair growth

D. All of the above

167. What is blood doping?

I. Infusing red blood cells to increase oxygen-carrying capacity

II. Taking erythropoietin (EPO) to increase red blood cell production

III. Injecting steroids to increase muscle mass and strength

A. I and II

B. I and III

C. II and III

D. I, II and III

168. Athletes may illegally use insulin for which of the following events?

A. Events that require high levels of endurance

B. Events that require strength

C. Events that require agility

D. Events that require flexibility

169. Which of the following is an example of progressive overload?

A. Lifting the same weight for the same number of repetitions in each workout

B. Increasing the weight lifted in each workout while keeping the number of repetitions constant

C. Decreasing the weight lifted in each workout while increasing the number of repetitions

D. Changing the exercises in each workout without altering the weight or repetitions

170. Which of the following is NOT a way to implement progressive overload?

A. Increasing the weight lifted

B. Increasing the number of repetitions performed

C. Decreasing the rest period between sets

D. Decreasing the intensity of the exercise

171. Which of the following repetition ranges is most appropriate for developing maximal strength?

A. 1-5 repetitions

B. 6-12 repetitions

C. 15-20 repetitions

D. 20+ repetitions

172. What does the first number in a tempo prescription signify?

A. Concentric phase duration

B. Eccentric phase duration

C. Isometric phase duration

D. Total time under tension

173. Which of the following is an example of a compound set?

A. Bench press followed by pull-ups

B. Squats followed by calf raises

C. Deadlifts followed by leg curls

D. Bench press followed by bicep curls

174. Which of the following best defines a drop set in resistance training?

A. Reducing the weight used during a set to allow for more repetitions

B. Alternating sets of two exercises for the same muscle group

C. Performing the same exercise at different tempos in one set

D. Using bands or chains to increase resistance during a set

175. When training and an athlete uses the drop set technique, what is the primary training goal?

A. Maximal strength

B. Muscular hypertrophy

C. Muscular endurance

D. Power development

176. Which of the following is an example of a compound exercise?

A. Bench press

B. Leg extension

C. Lateral raise

D. Tricep kickbacks

177. Which of the following training goals is best suited for using compound exercises?

A. Muscular endurance

B. Muscular hypertrophy

C. Maximal strength

D. Maximal Power

178. What is the Brzycki formula used for?

A. Estimating one-rep max

B. Calculating BMI

C. Measuring body fat percentage

D. Calculating resting heart rate

179. Which of the following statements best defines repetition maximum (RM)?

A. The maximum number of sets that can be performed in a given workout

B. The maximum number of repetitions that can be performed in a given set

C. The maximum weight that can be lifted for a given number of repetitions

D. The maximum amount of time that can be spent on a particular exercise

180. In which of the following grips are the palms facing each other, and the knuckles pointing forwards.?

A. Pronated grip

B. Supinated grip

C. Alternated grip

D. Neutral grip

181. Why is it recommended that athletes wear a weight belt during lifting?

A. To increase the amount of weight they can lift

B. To protect the lower back by increasing intra-abdominal pressure

C. To improve posture and form during lifts

D. To reduce the risk of developing muscle imbalances

182. Which of the following is an important requirement to be met when spotting over-the-face exercises?

A. The spotter should stand behind the lifter

B. The spotter should grip the lifter's forearms

C. The lifter should use a weightlifting belt

D. The lifter should have prior experience with the exercise

183. Which of these is not a correct technique used to perform the high-bar Olympic squat?

A. Lowering the body until the thighs are parallel to the ground.

B. Grasping the barbell with a narrow, overhand grip

C. Setting the barbell on the squat rack above chest height

D. Setting the feet shoulder-width apart, with the toes pointing slightly outward

184. During the snatch, what is the final position of the barbell?

A. Above the head with the arms fully extended

B. At shoulder height with the arms bent

C. At hip height with the arms extended

D. At knee height with the arms bent

185. What is the primary focus of Olympic weightlifting?

A. Explosive power

B. Cardiovascular endurance

C. Muscular endurance

D. Flexibility

186. Which of these statements accurately defines the difference between olympic weightlifting and plyometric exercise in terms of equipment use?

A. Olympic weightlifting utilizes weights, while plyometric exercise uses bodyweight

B. Plyometric exercise utilizes weights, while Olympic weightlifting uses bodyweight only

C. Olympic weightlifting uses heavier weights, while plyometric exercise utilizes lighter weights

D. Neither Olympic weightlifting nor plyometric exercise utilizes weights

187. What is the recommended height for depth jumps in plyometric exercise?

A. 15-32 inches

B. 16-42 inches

C. 25-54 inches

D. 30-56 inches

188. All of these are examples of ground-based free-exercise focused on training the core, except?

A. Leg press

B. Olympic lifts

C. Squats

D. Deadlifts

189. Which of these exercises uses variable resistance?

A. Bench press

B. Squats

C. Deadlifts

D. All of the options use variable resistance

190. Which of the following is an advantage of using variable resistance during training?

A. It reduces the risk of injury

B. It makes the exercise easier to perform

C. It increases muscle activation throughout the entire range of motion

D. It decreases the amount of time needed to complete a set

191. Which of the following exercises is most commonly performed using variable resistance?

A. Bench press

B. Bicep curls

C. Leg press

D. Lunges

192. The log lift is similar to which of the following exercises?

A. The snatch

B. The clean

C. The lift

D. The grip

193. Which of the following exercises is typically not associated with strongman training?

A. Bench press

B. Squat

C. Overhead press

D. Bicep curls

194. Which of the following is not a strongman exercise?

A. Deadlift

B. Tire flip

C. Farmer's walk

D. Box jump

195. Which of the following exercises should be performed last in a resistance training program?

A. Deadlift

B. Lat pulldown

C. Leg extension

D. Tricep Curl

196. What is the training volume for the barbell bench press exercise if you perform 6 sets of 10 reps with 190 pounds?

A. 5,700 pounds

B. 7,140 pounds

C. 11,400 pounds

D. 11,520 pounds

197: An athlete's estimated one-rep max for the squat is 300 pounds. What is the appropriate training load for the client if the program calls for 55% of their one-rep max?

A. 150 pounds

B. 165 pounds

C. 180 pounds

D. 195 pounds

198. Which of the following is a cause of fatigue during high-intensity exercise?

A. Depletion of muscle glycogen

B. Accumulation of lactate in the muscles

C. Increased core temperature

D. All of the above

199. Which of the following training methods is most effective at improving resistance to fatigue?

A. Low-intensity, long-duration exercise

B. High-intensity, short-duration exercise

C. Plyometric exercises

D. Circuit training

200. Which of the following factors can influence the magnitude and duration of the supercompensation effect?

A. Training intensity

B. Training frequency

C. Recovery time

D. All of the above

201. Which of these stages in designing a new strength and conditioning facility takes the longest time?

A. The pre-design phase

B. The design phase

C. Construction phase

D. Pre-operation phase

202. Which of the following is an important safety consideration when designing a strength and conditioning facility?

A. Providing adequate space for emergency responders

B. Installing high-intensity lighting for better visibility

C. Keeping the temperature at a constant level

D. Allowing clients to use equipment without supervision

203. The recommended ceiling height in a strength and conditioning facility is _____.

A. 8-10 ft

B. 12-14 ft

C. 16-22 ft

D. 24-28 ft

204. The aerobic area in a strength and conditioning facility houses all of the following equipment, except:

A. Treadmills

B. Rowing machines

C. Barbells and weights

D. Elliptical machines

205. An event linked to an injury that a court determines to be responsible is referred to as which of the following?

A. Negligence

B. Breach of Duty

C. Proximate Cause

D. Assumption of Risk

206. Which of the following is a fundamental movement pattern that involves moving weight away from the body?

A. Pull

B. Push

C. Hinge

D. Squat

207. Which of the following is a primary function of the biceps brachii muscle?

A. Elbow flexion

B. Elbow extension

C. Wrist flexion

D. Wrist extension

208. Which of the following is a common technique for improving power production in the lower body?

A. Resistance training with lower weights and high reps

B. Isometric training

C. Static stretching

D. Resistance training with low reps and heavy weights

209. Which of the following is a recommended technique for monitoring and adjusting training volume and intensity over time?

A. Periodization

B. Interval training

C. Circuit training

D. Super set

210. When designing a resistance training program, which of the following is recommended to prevent plateaus and improve long-term progress?

A. Varied exercise selection

B. Consistent exercise selection

C. Always using the same weight and reps

D. Training only one muscle group per workout

211. Which of the following is a common technique for improving endurance in aerobic activities?

A. Resistance training with low reps and heavy weights

B. High-intensity interval training (HIIT)

C. Isometric training

D. Plyometric training

212. What is the 300-yard shuttle run commonly used to measure?

A. Strength and power

B. Balance and coordination

C. Agility and anaerobic activity

D. Flexibility and range of motion

213. The lowering or muscle lengthening phase during an exertion is referred to as _____.

A. Eccentric

B. Concentric

C. Isomeric

D. Isocentric

214. Which type of validity is demonstrated by the high correlation between a 1 RM bench press and other accepted tests for measuring upper body strength?

A. Content validity

B. Construct validity

C. Concurrent validity

D. Predictive validity

215. During physical activity, the body loses electrolytes through sweat. Which of the following electrolytes is lost at the highest concentration during sweating?

A. Sodium

B. Magnesium

C. Phosphorus

D. Potassium

216. Which of the following are the best triglycerides recommended to include in a diet to reduce the risk of coronary artery disease?

A. Saturated fats

B. Monounsaturated fats

C. Polyunsaturated fats

D. Trans fats

217. What type of muscle action occurs when a muscle lengthens under tension, as in the lowering phase of a bicep curl?

A. Isometric

B. Eccentric

C. Concentric

D. Isotonic

218. Which of the following set-rep schemes is typically considered most effective for increasing muscle size?

A. 4 sets of 5 reps at 85% 1RM

B. 4 sets of 10 reps at 70% 1RM

C. 5 sets of 3 reps at 90% 1RM

D. 2 sets of 15 reps at 60% 1RM

219. When scheduling training sessions in a strength and conditioning facility, which of the following individuals would you give priority?

A. Those in preseason

B. Those in the off-season

C. Those in season

D. Women

220. How much work is required to lift a 170 kg barbell 2 m for 7 repetitions?

A. 23,324 J

B. 47,600 J

C. 35,520 J

D. 19,040 J

Test 2 Answers and Explanations

1. (C) Temporalis.

The temporalis, medial pterygoid, lateral pterygoid and masseter muscles are responsible for chewing or mastication. These muscles are connected to the mandible (lower jaw) and are among the strongest in the human body. Hence option C is correct.

2. (A) Fibrous joint.

The type of joint found in sutures and skulls is the fibrous joint. Fibrous joints are typically rigid and immovable and lack a joint cavity.

3. (B) Calcium and ATP.

Calcium and ATP must be present for myosin and actin cross bridges to function properly. Calcium ions bind to the regulatory protein troponin, which causes a change that exposes the myosin-binding sites on the actin filament. ATP, on the other hand, is needed to provide the energy necessary for the myosin heads to form cross-bridges with the actin filaments and to power the sliding of the filaments past each other during muscle contraction.

4. (A) Motor neurons.

There are three kinds of neurons: sensory, motor, and interneurons. Motor neurons are responsible for sending electrical signals from the brain to the muscles. Sensory neurons transmit signals from sensory organs, such as the eyes and ears, to the brain, while interneurons connect neurons within the brain and spinal cord. Interneurons do not have any role in neural transmission. Hence, option A is correct.

5. (C) They help in the development, maintenance, and repair of the synapse.

Perisynaptic Schwann cells in the Neuromuscular Junction help in the development, maintenance, and repair of the neuromuscular junction. Although Schwann cells indirectly contribute to muscle contraction, their primary role is in providing insulation and support to peripheral nerves. The breakdown of acetylcholine is primarily the function of acetylcholinesterase.

6. (B) The principle of inertia.

The principle of inertia measures how difficult it is to change an object's state of motion. According to this principle, the heavier the object, the more force is required to change its motion.

7. (C) Skeletal muscle.

Skeletal muscle makes up the majority of the total body weight in humans. In humans, skeletal muscles make up about 30 to 40% of the total body weight.

8. (B) It is anaerobic or oxygen independent.

The phosphagen system is anaerobic, or oxygen independent, as it does not require oxygen to resynthesize ATP. Option A is incorrect because this system does not use carbohydrates or fat to generate ATP. Instead, it uses creatine phosphate (CP) to generate ATP. Option C is incorrect because this system of producing energy is very handy during short-term, intense activities that need a large amount of energy. Option D is incorrect because there is a limited store of CP and ATP in the skeletal muscle. Also, fatigue occurs easily, making it hard for phosphagen to be used for endurance exercises.

9. (A) Epiglottis.

The epiglottis is the organ that prevents aspiration. It is a special flap of cartilage located at the opening of the larynx when a person swallows, thereby preventing food or liquid from entering the lungs. The pharynx, alveoli, and trachea are not directly involved in preventing aspiration.

10. (B) Loose connective tissue.

The loose connective tissue, also called areolar tissue, is the body's most abundant type of connective tissue. These tissues can be found in the outer part of the esophagus, blood vessels, nerves, and organs.

11. (A) Stroke volume.

Stroke volume is the volume of blood ejected out of the left ventricles during the systolic contraction. It is the difference between the end-diastolic volume and the end-systolic volume.

12. (C) Static stretching.

Static stretching, which involves holding a stretch for 15-30 seconds, is most appropriate during a cool-down as it helps improve flexibility, promotes relaxation, and aids in recovery.

13. (C) The SA node.

The SA node is also referred to as the pacemaker of the heart. The SA node is responsible for initiating each heartbeat and setting the heart's rhythm.

14. (A) Phosphagen.

The phosphagen energy system produces ATP at the fastest rate compared to the other energy systems listed. The phosphagen system relies on stored phosphocreatine (PCr) to rapidly regenerate ATP. Because this process does not require oxygen, it can produce ATP almost instantly.

15. (B) Cycling.

Low-impact exercises are those that place minimal stress on the joints, bones, and connective tissues of the body. Cycling would be considered a low-impact activity because it involves minimal joint stress.

16. (C) The principle of balance.

The principle of balance deals with the ability to control the body position in relation to the base of support of an object.

17. (B) Newton's first law of motion.

The principle of force-motion is based on Newton's first law of motion. It states that before motion can occur, some forces must act first.

18. (B) 206.

There are 206 bones in the adult human skeleton. Of these, there are 126 appendicular bones and 80 axial bones.

19. (B) Calcium influx.

When an action potential reaches the neuromuscular junction, it triggers the release of calcium ions from the sarcoplasmic reticulum in muscle cells. This influx of calcium ions causes the myosin heads to crosslink with the actin causing the muscle to contract.

20. (D) Pyramidalis.

The pyramidalis muscle is not found in the upper extremity as it is located in the lower abdomen. The trapezius muscle is located in the upper back, the brachioradialis muscle is located in the forearm, and the subclavius muscle is located under the collarbone, all in the upper extremity.

21. (B) Weight lifting.

Examples of isotonic exercise include walking, swimming, running, and cycling. Weight lifting is an example of an isometric exercise, and not isotonic. So, option B is the best answer.

22. (C) The hypothalamus and pituitary.

The main site of neuroendocrine interaction is the hypothalamus and pituitary.

23. (B) Vitamin B1.

People who regularly drink excess alcohol may find it hard to absorb vitamin B1 (thiamine) from their food. This may lead to vitamin B1 deficiency. Excessive alcohol consumption can also impair the ability of the intestine to absorb nutrients such as vitamin B12 and folate.

24. (C) 310-320 mg.

The Recommended dietary allowance (RDA) of magnesium for female adults aged 19 to 51 years is 310-320 mg daily for women.

25. (C) Achievement motivation.

Achievement motivation is characterized by an athlete's desire to compete or compare themselves with others. Intrinsic motivation is characterized by an inner drive to be good at something, while extrinsic motivation is driven by external sources or rewards, such as money, recognition, fame, or medals. Incentivized motivation is driven by a reward gotten for a particular action or the need to avoid action that attracts punishment.

26. (C) Flat bones.

The bones in the vertebrae and skull are irregular bones. Irregular bones are bones that have a complex shape and do not fit into the categories of long, short, or flat bones.

27. (B) Hammer curls.

The answer is hammer curls. Hammer curls primarily target the biceps. Lat pulldowns primarily work the latissimus dorsi, which is the large muscles of the back. Deadlifts, on the other hand, primarily work the glutes, hamstrings, and lower back muscles.

28. (B) Triceps.

The triceps muscle is an antagonist during a biceps curl. The biceps muscle flexes the elbow joint, while the triceps muscle extends the elbow joint.

29. (B) By reducing muscle fatigue.

Beta-alanine improves exercise performance primarily by reducing muscle fatigue. Beta-alanine may have some impact on other factors that can affect exercise performance, such as oxygen delivery and energy production. However, its primary mechanism of action is through the increase of muscle carnosine levels, which in turn helps to reduce muscle fatigue.

30. (A) Sagittal.

The sagittal plane is the anatomical plane that divides the body into left and right sections. The transverse plane divides the body into upper and lower sections, while the frontal or coronal plane divides the body into front and back sections.

31. (D) Muscle glycogen.

During a 400m run, the most probable limiting factor is muscle glycogen. This is because muscle glycogen is the primary fuel source for anaerobic metabolism. Hence as muscle glycogen stores become depleted, athletes may experience fatigue, decreased power output, and an inability to maintain their pace.

32. (A) The persistent eating of non-nutritive, non-food substances for at least a month.

Pica is an eating disorder defined as the persistent eating of non-nutritive, non-food substances for at least a month. This disorder involves the craving and consumption of non-food items, such as dirt, hair, ice, paper, or paint.

33. (B) SV = EDV – ESV.

The mathematical representation of stroke volume is SV = EDV – ESV

34. (B) Proteins.

Proteins are the most important nutrient for an athlete's recovery and tissue repair. Proteins help in the synthesis of new muscle tissue and support the immune system. Carbohydrates and fats are also important for athletes, as they provide the energy needed for exercise and aid in recovery; however, they do not play as critical a role in tissue repair as proteins do.

35. (B) Neurons.

The basic functional unit of the nervous system is referred to as a "neuron". Nephrons are the basic functional unit of the kidney, which are responsible for filtering blood and producing urine. Axons and dendrites are both parts of a neuron and are responsible for the transmission of signals.

36. (D) Use of compression garments.

Although all of the options listed can be helpful in promoting recovery in athletes, they do not have the same direct effect on neural signaling as compression garments.

37. (B). RMR = Body Weight x 10 + 22 x free fat mass(kg). The Cunningham equation is given as: RMR = 500+22 × {kg of free fat mass}.

38. (B) Negative reinforcement.

Negative reinforcement is the practice of eliminating a previously established consequence for an athlete's behavior following a successful performance. The goal of negative reinforcement is to increase the frequency of that behavior.

39. (B) Weight lifters.

The athletes with more type I fibers in their muscle cells are those who rely on aerobic endurance, as type I fibers are resistant to fatigue. Therefore, among the listed athletes, cross-country runners, endurance swimmers, and long-distance cyclists are more likely to have more type I fibers in their muscle cells. Weightlifters, on the other hand, rely on anaerobic power and strength, and therefore tend to have more type II fibers in their muscle cells. So, the correct answer is weight lifters.

40. (D) Calcium.

Calcium plays an important role in muscle contraction. When a muscle is stimulated to contract, calcium ions are released from the sarcoplasmic reticulum. After this, it binds to myosin and actin filaments leading to contraction. On the other hand, potassium, magnesium, and phosphorus do not have a direct role in muscle contraction like calcium does.

41. (C) Reflexibility.

Reflexibility is not a characteristic of muscle cells. The correct characteristics of muscle cells are excitability, contractility, and elasticity.

42. (B) 2.

When a molecule of glucose is broken down into pyruvate using glycolysis, only 2 molecules of ATP are produced in the process. However, additional ATP can be generated in subsequent stages of cellular respiration.

43. (D) Acetylcholine.

Acetylcholine is the chief neurotransmitter in the parasympathetic nervous system. It is involved in the transmission of nerve impulses at synapses.

44. (B) Legs bent at 90 degrees with feet on the ground.

The rectus abdominis muscle is most effectively activated during a crunch exercise when the legs are bent at 90 degrees with feet on the ground, as this position minimizes the involvement of the hip flexors.

45. (B) Oxidation of fats.

During the final phase of a marathon race, the body's primary source of ATP production shifts from aerobic metabolism to anaerobic metabolism due to the depletion of glycogen stores and a reduction in oxygen availability. Hence, the oxidation of fat provides the greatest supply of ATP in the final phase of a marathon race.

46. (D) mesocycle.

The mesocycle is a medium-length cycle, typically lasting several weeks to a few months, and is used to focus on specific training goals and objectives.

47. (A) Palms upward when grasping the bar.

In resistance training, a supinated grip describes a grip where the palms are facing upward and the knuckles are facing downward when grasping the bar. This grip places a greater emphasis on the biceps muscles and can be used for exercises such as chin-ups, bicep curls, and rows.

48. (A) Third-class lever.

A bicep curl involves a third-class lever. In a third-class lever, the effort (or force) is located between the load (or resistance) and the fulcrum. In a bicep curl, the biceps muscle applies the effort at the insertion point on the radius bone, the load is the weight of the dumbbell or barbell being lifted, and the fulcrum is the elbow joint.

49. (C) Eosinophils.

Eosinophils are white blood cells that take part in allergic inflammatory reactions. Lymphocytes are a type of white blood cells that are important for the immune system to respond to allergens and parasites. Neutrophils are the most abundant type of white blood cells and play a key role in the immune response to infection.

50. (A) Bodyweight

Push-ups, pull-ups, and chin-ups are examples of bodyweight exercises. Bodyweight exercises are exercises that use the weight of the body itself as resistance, rather than external weights or equipment.

51. (C) The log-lift.

The log-lift is not one of the main techniques for tire flipping. The three techniques commonly used techniques for flipping tires include the sumo, backlift style, and shoulders-against-the-tire technique. The log-lift is a technique used in strongman competitions.

52. (C) Circuit training.

Circuit training involves doing a sequence of exercises back-to-back without rest, repeated multiple times. In circuit training, you perform a set of exercises for a certain amount of time or a certain number of repetitions before moving on to the next exercise in the circuit. Option B, progressive overload, refers to gradually increasing the demands on your muscles in order to continue making progress. On the other hand, high intensity training involves performing exercises at a very high level of intensity for short periods of time, while isometric training involves holding a static contraction in a particular muscle or muscle group without any movement. Hence, option C is the correct answer.

53. (D) Guided imagery.

The correct answer is guided imagery. This technique involves focusing on calming mental images and sensations, such as imagining oneself in a peaceful setting, to promote relaxation and reduce stress. Option A, Progressive Muscle Relaxation, involves tensing and relaxing different muscle groups in the body to promote relaxation and reduce physical tension. Option B, Autogenic Training, involves focusing on physical sensations such as warmth and heaviness in different parts of the body to promote relaxation. Option C, Deep Breathing Exercises, involve focusing on slow, deep breathing to promote relaxation and reduce stress. Hence, option D is the correct answer.

54. (C) NEEDs analysis.

The needs analysis involves identifying the essential characteristics required for the athlete, the sport, or a combination of both. One important component of the NEEDs analysis is the injuries analysis. The injury analysis involves finding out the common injuries in that sport and position, how frequently these injuries occur, predisposing factors to these injuries, and total injuries every year.

55. (A) Assistance exercise.

The barbell biceps curl is classified as an assistance exercise. Assistance exercises are movements that target specific muscle groups or assist in the development of other exercises, especially compound exercises. The barbell biceps curl specifically targets the biceps muscles, which are located on the front of the upper arm.

56. (D) Suspended wood floor.

A suspended wood floor is best suited for plyometric training. Plyometric training often involves explosive and high-impact movements that can put a lot of stress on the joints and connective tissues. However, using surfaces such as a suspended wood floor, can help absorb some of the shock and reduce the risk of injury.

57. (C.) Impulse.

Impulse is the product of force and time, and it represents the change in an object's momentum that results from the application of a force over a period of time. Velocity is a measure of the speed and direction of an object, while acceleration is the rate of change of velocity over time. Momentum is the product of an object's mass and velocity. Hence, the correct option is Impulse.

58. (A) Powerlifting.

Short rest periods are not recommended for powerlifting exercises. This is because longer rest periods are necessary to allow for adequate recovery between sets. Powerlifting exercises, such as the squat, bench press, and deadlift, require a high level of muscular force and often involve lifting heavy loads. As a result, longer rest periods of 2-5 minutes between sets are typically recommended to allow for the recovery of the muscles and nervous system. Although weight lifting exercises, such as the clean and jerk or snatch, depending on if they are performed at high intensities or with heavier loads, can also require longer rest periods. Hence, the best option is A.

59. (A) 6.

When designing a strength and conditioning facility, mirrors should be positioned at least 6 inches away from equipment and 20 inches above the floor to avoid damage from dropped weights or plates.

60. (B). Muscle hypertrophy

An athlete performing 3 to 4 sets of 8-10 repetitions of the same exercise is most likely trying to increase muscle hypertrophy, which refers to an increase in muscle size. The recommended range of repetitions for hypertrophy training is typically 8-12 reps per set, which is consistent with the athlete's training program of 3-4 sets of 8-10 reps.

61. (B) Concrete.

Plyometric exercises involve explosive jumping and hopping movements that create high impact forces on the body and the ground. However, concrete floors are hard surfaces that do not absorb shock, which can increase the risk of injury to the joints and bones of the lower body. Hence, they are not recommended for plyometric exercise. On the other hand, grass fields, suspended floors, and rubber mats are recommended for plyometric exercises as they offer some level of shock absorption and can help reduce the impact forces on the body. So, option B is correct.

62. (D) Momentum.

Momentum is defined as the relationship between mass and velocity. The greater an object's mass and velocity, the greater its momentum.

63. (C) To promote peak performance.

The primary purpose of tapering before a competition is to promote peak performance by reducing the training volume and allowing the body to fully recover and adapt to the previous training.

64. (B) Resistance phase.

During the resistance phase of the General Adaptation Syndrome (GAS), the body adapts to the training stimulus and returns to a state of equilibrium. This phase is characterized by improved performance and increased physiological capacity, as the body adapts to meet the demands of the training program.

65. (C) Off-season.

The off-season is the period during which a coach should focus on improving weaknesses and maintaining the strengths of athletes. This phase is considered the preparation period and provides an opportunity for athletes to focus on their training and development.

66. (C) Oxidative system.

The oxidative or aerobic system is the energy system mainly utilized in endurance cycling. This system uses oxygen to produce energy from the breakdown of carbohydrates, fats, and proteins. It is a very suitable energy source for endurance activities such as cycling, which require sustained effort over an extended period of time. On the other hand, the glycolytic system and phosphagen system are used for shorter-duration, high-intensity activities such as sprinting or weightlifting. The concentric system is not an energy system.

67. (B) 68- 78°F.

The temperature for a strength and conditioning facility should be kept between 68°F to 78°F (20-25 °C). This temperature range provides a comfortable environment for athletes to exercise in without being too hot or too cold.

68. (C) Diuretics.

Diuretics are often used as a masking agent to avoid detection of another banned substance in sports. Erythropoietin is majorly used in blood doping to improve endurance and reduce fatigue. Creatine can help to improve strength, power, and muscle mass, while ephedrine is a stimulant that can increase energy, focus, and performance.

69. (B) Decrease carbohydrate intake.

During a period of reduced training volume or tapering, an athlete should decrease their carbohydrate intake to match the decreased energy demands. Protein and fat intake should remain relatively consistent to support muscle maintenance and overall health.

70. (A). The number of years a person has been consistently training in a structured and supervised program. Training age is typically used in the context of strength training to refer to the number of years a person has been consistently training in a structured and supervised program. It measures a person's body's experience and adaptation to strength training.

71. (B) Head.

During seated or supine bench exercises, the head is not one of the five points of contact. The five points of contact are typically the left foot, right foot, buttocks, left hand, and right hand, or a variation, depending on the exercise. Certain exercises may also include the lower back as a point of contact. Hence, the best answer is B.

72. (B) Hips higher than knees, back straight, toes pointing forward.

The proper deadlift form is hips higher than knees, back straight, and toes pointing forward. This position is also known as the "hip hinge" position.

73. (D). None of the above.

All the factors mentioned (genetic predisposition to mental health issues, injuries or chronic pain, and performance anxiety) can contribute to mental health issues in athletes.

74. (C) Calcium.

Athletes who avoid dairy may struggle to meet their calcium requirements, as dairy products are one of the main sources of dietary calcium.

75. (A) Binge eating followed by purging.

Bulimia nervosa is characterized by binge eating followed by purging. People suffering from bulimia nervosa frequently experience binge eating episodes in which they consume an unusually large amount of food in a short period of time and feel a lack of control over their eating. Purging, which can include self-induced vomiting, the misuse of laxatives, diuretics, or enemas, or other inappropriate compensatory behaviors to prevent weight gain, is typically followed by these episodes.

76. (C) Deadlift.

The deadlift is usually considered the best exercise to perform first in a resistance training session because it involves the most muscle groups and requires the most energy.

77. (C) Recommend that the athlete seek advice from a knowledgeable nutritionist or dietitian.

When asked which brand of creatine a 17-year-old athlete should use, a strength and conditioning coach should recommend that the athlete consult with a knowledgeable nutritionist or dietitian.

78. (B) Consume 400 additional kilocalories and 128 g of protein.

A weightlifter should consume an additional 400 kilocalories and 128 grams of protein per day to gain 4 kg of lean body mass. This will result in a calorie surplus, which can promote muscle growth when combined with resistance training. The recommended protein intake for muscle growth is 1.6-2.2 grams per kilogram of body weight per day. Therefore, the weightlifter must consume more protein to support muscle growth, in addition to increasing her overall calorie intake. This answer is based on estimations.

79. (B) Caffeine.

Caffeine is a banned substance that is commonly used to increase alertness and reduce fatigue. Creatine is used to enhance athletic performance and increase muscle mass. Furosemide is a diuretic drug and may be used to mask the effect of other banned drug substances. Nitric oxide is sometimes used as a dietary supplement to enhance athletic performance.

80. (D) Growth hormone.

Growth hormone is a hormone that the body produces naturally. Although it is commonly used to treat certain medical conditions, it is also abused by athletes in order to increase muscle mass and strength. Athletes use insulin to increase muscle growth or improve performance. The thyroid is used by athletes to increase metabolism and energy expenditure. Athletes may use cortisol-like drugs, called corticosteroids, to reduce inflammation, improve recovery, or enhance performance. The best option is D.

81. (D) To provide a stable foundation for lifting heavy loads.

The Valsalva maneuver is a technique used during weightlifting exercises to stabilize the spine and increase intra-abdominal pressure, which can help the person lift heavier weights. Hence the best option is D. The Valsalva maneuver can be used to help stabilize the spine and increase intra-abdominal pressure, which can help the person lift heavier weights.

82. (A) Increase the risk of injury if the load or exercise is done too frequently.

Although using progressive overload in a resistance training program can be an effective way to increase strength and muscle mass, it can also increase the risk of injury if the load or exercise is performed too frequently or incorrectly. As a result, it is important to gradually increase the load and intensity while maintaining proper form and allowing enough time for rest and recovery.

83. (C) Tempo.

Tempo in strength training refers to the rate or speed at which a resistance exercise is performed. It is usually expressed as a series of numbers that represent the time spent during each phase of the exercise. Reps refer to the number of times an exercise is repeated during a set. Sets refer to the number of cycles of repetitions completed during an exercise session. Also, velocity refers to the rate of displacement or speed of movement during an exercise. So, the correct answer is C–Tempo.

84. (B) The portion of the exercise where the muscle lengthens.

The portion of the exercise where the muscle lengthens is known as the eccentric phase. The concentric phase, on the other hand, is the portion of the exercise where the muscle shortens or contracts. Hence, option B is correct.

85. (B) By keeping the tendon away from the center of rotation at the knee.

The patella keeps the tendon away from the center of rotation at the knee, reducing friction and wear on the tendon. It also helps distribute force evenly across the knee joint, reducing stress and strain on the joint during activity

86. (A) 158-169 bpm.

Calculate the maximum heart rate (HRmax): HRmax = 220 – age

Calculate the heart rate reserve (HRR): HRR = HRmax - resting heart rate

Determine the desired intensity: For a target intensity of 60% to 70%, the desired intensity can be expressed as 0.6 × HRR to 0.7 × HRR

Calculate the target heart rate: Target heart rate = resting heart rate + (desired intensity × HRR)

For a 40-year-old with a resting heart rate of 68:

HRmax = 220 - 40 = 180 bpm

HRR = 180 - 68 = 112

Desired intensity = 0.8 × 112 to 0.9 × 112 = 90 to 101

Target heart rate = 68 + 90 to 68 + 101 = 158 to 169

87. (C) Box drills.

Box drills are an example of a plyometric exercise. Plyometric exercises are designed to increase power and explosiveness in the muscles, and they involve jumping or hopping movements. Box drills involve jumping on and off a platform or box, and they require explosive power from the leg muscles. Bicep curl and tricep extension are both isolation exercises that focus on the arm muscles. Lat pulldown is a compound exercise that works the back and arm muscles. Neither of the three options involve explosive movements that are characteristic of plyometric exercises. Hence, option C is correct.

88. (C) With a mixed grip.

The barbell should be gripped with a mixed grip when performing a sumo deadlift, which means one hand should have an overhand grip and the other hand should have an underhand grip. The overhand grip on one hand and the underhand grip on the other hand keep the bar balanced during the lift. A narrow, overhand grip or a narrow, underhand grip may not be stable enough for the lift, whereas a wide, overhand grip may be too wide and uncomfortable for the lifter.

89. (A) Agility training.

Agility training is used to develop the ability to change direction quickly. Plyometric training can improve power, explosiveness, and speed, but it doesn't specifically focus on changing direction quickly. Speed training can increase running speed, but it doesn't necessarily help with changing direction quickly. And the same goes for strength training, so the best answer is A.

90. (B) To identify areas where the athlete needs improvement.

The primary purpose of a needs analysis in sports training is to determine the athlete's current physical abilities and identify areas where the athlete needs improvement.

91. (C) Dietary preferences.

The needs analysis in sports training evaluates the athlete's current movement patterns, injury history, exercise history, and sport-specific requirements. Dietary preferences, on the other hand, are not typically included in a needs analysis, as they are not directly related to an athlete's physical abilities and performance in the same way that movement patterns, exercise history, and injury history are.

92. (A) Compound exercises before isolation exercises.

When performing a resistance training workout, the recommended exercise order is typically to begin with compound exercises that target multiple muscle groups before progressing to isolation exercises that target specific muscle groups. This is due to the fact that compound exercises are more complex and require more energy and coordination.

93. (B) Z-Drill.

All of the options given (A-Skip, Fast Feet, and Sprint Resistance) except Z-Drill are examples of speed drills. Z-Drill is a type of agility drill that involves changing direction and speed in response to visual or verbal cues.

94. (B) Dismissal from the facility for one week.

The discipline system in place involves a tiered penalty system. In the event of a first offense, a verbal warning will be issued by the staff. A second offense results in dismissal from the facility for one day, with the offense being recorded. A third offense will result in a one-week dismissal from the facility. Further offenses will incur stricter penalties. Hence, the correct answer is B.

95. (C) Russian twists.

Russian twists are rotational exercises that primarily target core muscles, such as the transverse abdominis, which is in charge of spinal stability and rotation. As a result, Russian twists are primarily used to strengthen the transverse plane. Bicep curls and shoulder press exercises are performed primarily in the sagittal plane, which is the plane that divides the body into left and right halves. Lunges are primarily performed in the sagittal and frontal planes, which divide the body into front and back halves.

96. (A). 490 W

Work = force x distance work = 100 kg x 9.8 m/s^2 x 2 m work = 1960 joules

To find the power output, divide the work done by the time it took to do it:

Power = work / time power = 1960 J / 4 s power = 490 watts

97. (C) Testosterone.

Testosterone is the primary hormone responsible for stimulating muscle protein synthesis, which leads to increased muscle mass and strength. This anabolic hormone plays a crucial role in the body's ability to recover and adapt to resistance training.

98. (D) Leg extension.

The leg extension primarily targets the quadriceps muscle group, which is responsible for knee extension. This exercise isolates the quadriceps muscles and can be used to build strength and endurance in the front of the thigh.

99. (C) Narrow, overhand grip.

The recommended grip for a barbell bench press is a narrow, overhand grip, whereas a narrow, underhand grip and mixed grip are not advised.

100. (D) Rate of force development.

The primary factor that determines an athlete's ability to generate force in executing movement techniques is the rate of force development. The rate of force development refers to how quickly an athlete can increase their force production, and it is influenced by factors such as neuromuscular efficiency, muscle fiber type, and training history.

101. (C) Supercompensation is a process by which the body overcompensates for the stress of exercise, resulting in increased levels of strength and endurance.

102. (C) Narrow, overhand grip.

The proper grip for the barbell when performing a high-bar Olympic squat is a narrow, overhand grip. This grip allows for better control and stability of the barbell during the lift and also helps to engage the upper back muscles to maintain a straight and upright posture. Using a wide grip can cause the barbell to roll forward on the shoulders, making it difficult to maintain proper form and balance.

103. (D) All of the above.

All of the options are correct. Understanding organizational trends and best practices in strength and conditioning can help a strength and conditioning specialist stay current with the latest research, implement best practices in their program, and provide better training for their athletes. By keeping up with the latest trends and practices, a specialist can develop more effective training programs and provide their athletes with the best possible training experience.

104. (D) To adapt the training program to the specific demands of the sport and optimize performance.

The goal of incorporating sport seasons into periodization cycles is to adapt the training program to the specific demands of the sport and optimize performance. By planning and organizing the training program around the competitive season, the athlete can peak at the right time and perform at their best. This entails adjusting the training goals and objectives, as well as the training intensity, volume, and frequency, to match the demands of the sport during each phase of the periodization cycle.

105. (B) Acknowledgment of inherent risk in participating and choosing to participate anyway.

Assumption of risk is the acknowledgment of inherent risk in participating and choosing to participate anyway.

106. (D) Improve short-term, high-intensity performance.

Creatine supplementation primarily serves to improve short-term, high-intensity performance by increasing the availability of creatine phosphate, which helps rapidly regenerate ATP during high-intensity activities.

107. (D) His initial caffeine levels.

During the tempo run, his initial caffeine levels have no effect on his heart rate. While caffeine is a stimulant that can increase heart rate during exercise, the runner's initial caffeine levels may not significantly impact their heart rate during a tempo run, especially if caffeine consumption was not recent. The intensity of the exercise, as well as individual factors such as age, gender, and fitness level, all influence the heart rate during exercise. The duration of the exercise session, the runner's state of training, and the runner's gender can all affect heart rate during a tempo run.

108. (D) Both A and C.

The primary goal of a dynamic warm-up is to increase muscle temperature and blood flow while also activating the central nervous system. This type of warm-up prepares the body for high-intensity exercise by improving joint mobility, muscle elasticity, and neuromuscular function.

109. (D) Hydration status.

Factors that affect an individual's flexibility include muscle temperature, joint structure, and age. Although hydration status is essential for overall health and exercise performance, it has a minimal direct impact on flexibility.

110. (A) I and II.

Resistance training benefits include increased muscle mass and strength, as well as bone density maintenance. As a result, the answer is I and II. While resistance training can improve muscle flexibility, it may not necessarily improve joint flexibility. Hence, option III is incorrect. While some resistance training exercises require equipment, such as dumbbells or resistance bands, there are many exercises that can be done with just your own body weight, such as push-ups, squats, and lunges. Hence, resistance training can also be performed at home without equipment. So, option IV is incorrect.

111. (A) 25lbs.

To find the weight that should be used with the 20 lb. resistance band:

Previous 10RM weight = 45 lbs. Resistance provided by band = 20 lbs.

Weight with resistance band = Previous 10RM weight - Resistance provided by band.

Weight with resistance band = 45 lbs. - 20 lbs.

Weight with resistance band = 25 lbs.

Therefore, the weight that should be used is 20 lb. resistance band is 25 lbs.

112. (C) Body weight, age (years), and free fat mass (FFM).

The variables used in Cunningham's equation to calculate RMR are body weight, free fat mass (FFM), and age. Therefore, the correct answer is weight, age, and free fat mass (kg).

113. (D) Increased capillary density.

The physiological adaptation that leads to an increase in the amount of oxygen transported into the blood for the muscle's use during aerobic activity is an increase in capillary density. When there is an increase in capillary density, it allows for greater diffusion of oxygen into the blood, resulting in an increased amount of oxygen being transported to the muscle for use during aerobic activity.

114. (B) His gender.

Muscle fatigue is affected by several factors, including the number of sets performed, the state of training, and initial hydration levels. Gender, however, is not a direct determinant of muscle fatigue during exercise. Hence. Option B is correct.

115. (D) Intra-rater reliability.

The type of reliability test used to measure the consistency of scores across raters is intra-rater reliability. This test compares the similarity of scores from different raters or different test forms.

116. (C) Excitability.

The characteristic of muscles that depicts their ability to react to stimulus is excitability. Excitability, also known as irritability, is the ability of muscle cells to respond to a stimulus, such as an electrical impulse or a chemical signal. Contractility is the ability of a muscle to contract or shorten in response to a stimulus, while extensibility refers to the ability of a muscle to be stretched or extended without being damaged. Elasticity is the ability of a muscle to return to its original shape after being stretched or contracted. Hence, Option C is the correct answer.

117. (B) Tendon.

Tendons connect the skeletal muscles to the bones. Tendons are tough and flexible bands of connective tissue that connect muscle to bone and transmit the force generated by muscle contraction to produce movement.

118. (D) Quadratus femoris.

Quadratus femoris is not a muscle found in the upper extremities. It is actually a muscle located in the posterior hip region. The other three muscles mentioned (biceps brachii, triceps brachii, and deltoid) are all muscles found in the upper extremities.

119. (B) Gluteus ilium.

The muscle that is not part of the glutes is "gluteus ilium." There is no muscle named "gluteus ilium." However, the ilium is one of the three bones that make up the pelvis. The three muscle that makes up the glute include gluteus maximus, gluteus minimus, and gluteus medius.

120. (C) type IIB.

Splinters have an abundance of type IIB fibers. Type IIB fibers produce high force.

121. (B) Hyaline.

Cartilaginous joints are composed solely of either hyaline cartilage or fibrocartilage. So, the correct option is "Hyaline."

122. (B) Increased protein synthesis.

Skeletal muscle adapts to mechanical overload through a process called muscle hypertrophy, which involves increased protein synthesis and the addition of new muscle fibers to the affected area. This leads to an increase in muscle size and strength. Decreased mitochondrial density, increased muscle fiber atrophy, and decreased myofibrillar hypertrophy are not typical adaptations to mechanical overload. Hence, option B is the correct answer.

123. (C) Improved aerobic metabolism.

Endurance training is most likely to target and improve aerobic metabolism. This type of training leads to adaptations that improve the body's ability to use oxygen efficiently, including increased capillary density, improved mitochondrial function, and increased production of enzymes involved in oxidative metabolism. Endurance training is less likely to target increases in muscle size or myofibrillar protein synthesis, although it may still have some impact on these adaptations. Decreased mitochondrial density is not an adaptation that would be targeted or desired with endurance training.

124. (A) Thin.

Short bones are typically cube-shaped and appear flattened. They are generally small, with a layer of compact bone on the outside and cancellous bone on the inside. Short bones are not typically thin; rather, they are thick and sturdy. Short bones can be slightly curved depending on their location in the body and function. As a result, "thin" is an incorrect characteristic of short bones.

125. (A) It appears as a large uniocular lipid droplet under a microscope.

Under the microscope, the brown adipose tissue is seen as multiple small lipid droplets. Hence, option A is incorrect. All of the other options are correct. The main function of BAT is to generate heat by consuming energy reserves in the body through a process called thermogenesis. It is often found in infants and decreases with age, which is why it is sometimes referred to as "baby fat."

126. (B) Blood.

Blood is the connective tissue that lacks fibers. Unlike the other types of connective tissues mentioned, blood does not contain fibers such as collagen or elastin. Instead, blood is composed of various types of cells and a liquid extracellular matrix called plasma.

127. (A) The Resistive force is less than the applied force.

When the mechanical advantage is greater than 1, the resistive force is less than the applied force. Therefore, the correct statement is "The Resistive force is less than the applied force."

128. (C) Smaller individuals may have an advantage in strength-to-weight ratio.

Smaller individuals may have an advantage in strength-to-weight ratio. This is because muscle strength is not only determined by size but also by factors such as muscle fiber type, neuromuscular efficiency, and training status.

129. (B) High-intensity, low-volume strength training.

High-intensity, low-volume strength training is most effective for increasing muscle size and strength. This type of training involves using heavy weights for fewer repetitions with adequate rest periods between sets. This type of training stresses the muscles to a greater extent, causing them to adapt and become stronger and larger over time.

130. (C) Shoulders.

Overhead lifts pose the greatest risk to the shoulders. The shoulder joint is a complex joint with a high degree of mobility, which makes it vulnerable to injury during overhead lifts if proper form and technique are not used.

131. (A) Warm up with heavy weights.

Warming up with heavy weights is not a good way for athletes to reduce their risk of injury. Before beginning any exercise or sports activity, a proper warm-up should be performed, but heavy weights should not be used. To prepare the body for more intense activity, a warm-up should include light aerobic activity, dynamic stretching, and mobility exercises.

132. (B) Metabolism.

The sum of all chemical reactions in a biological system is referred to as metabolism. These reactions include anabolic (molecule-building) and catabolic (molecule-breaking) reactions, as well as all other chemical processes that occur in cells and organisms to sustain life.

133. (C) Interval training.

Interval training targets a specific body area by alternating between periods of exercise and rest. This type of training involves alternating between high-intensity exercise and low-intensity or rest periods, which can be designed to target specific muscle groups or areas of the body.

134. (A) Diaphragm.

During normal breathing, the diaphragm is primarily in charge of inhalation. It is a dome-shaped muscle located at the bottom of the rib cage that separates the thoracic cavity from the abdominal cavity. When it contracts, it flattens and moves downward, increasing the volume of the thoracic cavity and drawing air into the lungs. The external intercostals also contribute to inhalation by elevating the ribs and expanding the chest cavity, but the diaphragm is the primary muscle involved in normal breathing.

135. (C) Nasal cavity.

The nasal cavity is in charge of filtering and warming the incoming air. When we breathe in through our noses, the air travels through the nasal cavity, which is lined with tiny hairs called cilia and mucous membranes that help filter out dust, dirt, and other particles. The nasal cavity also warms and humidifies the air as it passes through, which helps to protect the respiratory system's delicate tissues.

136. (D) 55%.

Blood is made up of approximately 55% plasma. Plasma is the liquid component of blood that carries various substances, such as proteins, hormones, electrolytes, and waste products, throughout the body. The other components of blood include red blood cells (which make up about 45% of blood volume), white blood cells, and platelets.

137. (D) Spleen.

The spleen is not a component of the cardiovascular system. The cardiovascular system consists of the heart, blood vessels, and blood, while the spleen is part of the lymphatic system. The spleen plays a role in filtering the blood, removing old or damaged red blood cells, and helping to fight infections.

138. (C) Myocardium.

The name of the muscular layer of the heart is the myocardium. The endocardium is the innermost layer of the heart. The pericardium is the outermost layer of the heart. The epicardium is the inner layer of the pericardium that is in contact with the outer surface of the heart.

139. (D) Pulmonary vein.

The structure that receives oxygenated blood from the lungs and drains it into the left atrium is the pulmonary vein. The superior vena cava is a large vein that carries deoxygenated blood from the upper body and arms to the right atrium of the heart. The Inferior vena cava is a large vein that carries deoxygenated blood from the lower body and legs to the right atrium of the heart. The pulmonary artery is a large artery that carries deoxygenated blood from the right ventricle of the heart to the lungs, where the blood becomes oxygenated.

140. (C) Atria.

The atria are not a part of the cardiac conduction system. The cardiac conduction system consists of the sinoatrial (SA) node, atrioventricular (AV) node, bundle of HIS, Purkinje fibers and Ventricles.

141. (A) Atria first, then the ventricles.

The correct sequence of the movement of the electrical impulse generated by the Sinoatrial (SA) node is the atria first, then the ventricles.

142. (B) Diastole.

The period of time during the cardiac cycle when the heart is relaxed and filled with blood is called diastole. Systole is the period during the cardiac cycle when the heart is contracting, and blood is being pumped out of the heart into the arteries. The ejection phase is a part of the systole where the heart is actively ejecting blood from the left ventricle into the aorta. The preload refers to the amount of blood in the ventricles at the end of diastole, just before the systole begins. Hence, the correct answer is B.

143. (D) 140/90mmHg.

Out of the options given, the figure that depicts high blood pressure is 140/90mmHg. Blood pressure is considered high if the systolic pressure is consistently at or above 140 mmHg, or if the diastolic pressure is consistently at or above 90 mmHg. Considering the other options given, 90/60mmHg is considered to be hypotension (low blood pressure), 120/80mmHg is normal, and 130/90mmHg is classified as stage 1 hypertension.

144. (B) Extension of the elbow joint.

The primary function of the triceps brachii muscle is to extend the elbow joint. This muscle is activated during pushing movements, such as a push-up or bench press, as well as during triceps-specific exercises like the triceps extension.

145. (B) Enhanced proprioception and neuromuscular control.

Incorporating balance and stability exercises into a strength and conditioning program can enhance proprioception and neuromuscular control. This improved body awareness and control can contribute to better overall movement quality, injury prevention, and performance in various sports and activities.

146. (B) Increased stroke volume.

Athletes who engage in regular aerobic exercise typically have lower resting heart rates than sedentary individuals. One of the ways this occurs is through an increase in stroke volume, which is the amount of blood pumped out of the heart with each beat. Hence, option B is the best answer.

147. (A) Increased cardiac output.

Increased stroke volume directly results in increased cardiac output, which is the amount of blood pumped by the heart per minute.

148. (B) I and II.

An increase in myoglobin levels is one of the major reasons why oxygen uptake increases during exercise/training. During exercise, as oxygen consumption increases, the demand for oxygen by the working muscles also increases. The increase in myoglobin levels within the muscle fibers helps to facilitate the delivery of oxygen to the mitochondria, where it is used to produce energy for muscle contraction. Regular endurance exercise can stimulate the production of additional red blood cells, resulting in an increase in hemoglobin levels, which in turn can increase the oxygen-carrying capacity of the blood. However, increased protein synthesis is not a direct reason why oxygen uptake increases during exercise/training. Hence, the correct answer is I and II.

149. (D) People who have no prior training experience.

When individuals are new to training or have little prior training experience, they have a greater potential for adaptation than those who have been training for several years. This is because at the beginning of training, the body is not used to the stress of exercise. Therefore, even small increases in activity can lead to significant gains in strength or endurance.

150. (D) All of the above.

Active recovery, cryotherapy, and compression garments are all effective recovery methods for reducing delayed onset muscle soreness.

151. (C) Incorporating plyometric exercises.

Plyometric exercises, such as jump squats and box jumps, involve high-intensity muscle contractions and explosive movements. They can help athletes improve their power by increasing neuromuscular coordination, increasing the rate of force production, and increasing muscle fiber recruitment.

152. (C) Varying the type and intensity of exercises.

Resistance training can cause muscle damage, leading to delayed onset muscle soreness (DOMS). To promote recovery, it is important to allow adequate time for rest and recovery between resistance training sessions. Varying the type and intensity of exercises can help prevent overuse injuries and reduce the risk of plateaus. Hence, option C is correct.

153. (A) Active recovery.

Active recovery is an effective recovery method for promoting muscle repair and reducing inflammation. Cryotherapy, which involves exposing the body to cold temperatures, can also be effective in reducing inflammation and promoting recovery; however, it is majorly used for acute injuries. Static stretching and debriefing can be useful in improving flexibility but they are not as effective as active recovery for promoting muscle repair and reducing inflammation.

154. (D) All the options are important.

All the options listed play a significant role in ensuring that patients with disabilities receive the same quality of care as patients without disabilities. Modified facilities, adapted equipment, and personal assistants or interpreters are essential to ensure that patients with disabilities can access and receive the care they need without facing any barriers.

155. (A) Perceived competence.

Perceived competence refers to an individual's belief in their ability to successfully perform a task or achieve a goal. Perceived competence is a key component of achievement motivation because individuals who perceive themselves as competent are more likely to be motivated to engage in tasks and strive for success. Anxiety, social support, and internal locus of control may also play a role in motivation and achievement, but not to a great extent as perceived competence.

156. (C) Feelings of sadness or anxiety.

Psychological symptoms that indicate a mental health issue in athletes include anxiety, insomnia or hypersomnia, feelings of sadness, hopelessness etc. Poor coordination and balance, reduced performance, increased heart rate, and blood pressure are physical symptoms related to sports injury.

157. (C) Chronic pain or injury.

Chronic pain or injury is a potential risk factor for mental health issues in athletes. Chronic pain or injury can lead to feelings of frustration, helplessness, and despair, which can contribute to mental health issues such as anxiety and depression.

158. (C) Fats.

Fats provide the highest amount of energy per gram among the macronutrients. One gram of fat contains 9 calories, while one gram of protein and carbohydrates contains 4 calories each. Fiber is not a macronutrient and does not provide energy as it is not digested by the body.

159. (A) Vitamin D.

Vitamin D is a micronutrient that is important for bone health and can be found in dairy products, leafy greens, and fortified foods. Vitamin D is necessary for the absorption of calcium, which is a key mineral for bone health. Iron, zinc, and magnesium are important micronutrients for various bodily functions, but they are not directly related to bone health.

160. (C) Monounsaturated fats.

Monounsaturated fat is referred to as a healthy source of dietary fat, while saturated fats and trans fats are considered unhealthy. Monounsaturated fats can be found in foods such as avocados, nuts, seeds, and olive oil. They can help lower bad cholesterol levels and reduce the risk of heart disease.

161. (B) Pica.

Pica is an eating disorder in which an individual craves and eats non-food items, such as paper, chalk, or dirt.

162. (C) 7.

1g of alcohol contains approximately 7 Kcals of energy.

163. (A) 223 calories.

I g of protein= 4 calories

I gram carbohydrate= 4 calories

I g of fats= 9 calories

Protein: 40 grams x 4 calories/gram = 160 calories

Carbs: 10 grams x 4 calories/gram = 40 calories

Fat: 2.5 grams x 9 calories/gram = 22.5 calories

Total calories in the protein bar = 160 + 40 + 22.5 = 222.5 calories.

Therefore, the protein bar will have approximately 223 calories.

164. (B) During exercise.

The best time to drink fluids during exercise to avoid dehydration is during exercise. Drinking fluids while exercising helps to replace fluids lost through sweating and maintain optimal hydration levels, which is critical for maintaining performance and avoiding dehydration-related issues.

165. (B) Endurance performance.

Beta-alanine is commonly used as a supplement to enhance endurance performance. Beta-alanine is an amino acid that is used to produce carnosine, which is stored in the muscles and helps to regulate acid-base balance during high-intensity exercise.

166. (D) All of the above.

All of the above are common side effects of anabolic steroid use in women. All of the above are common side effects of anabolic steroid use in women. Anabolic steroids are synthetic hormones that are used to promote muscle growth and improve athletic performance. In women, the use of anabolic steroids can lead to a range of masculinizing side effects, including deepening of the voice (hoarseness), decreased breast size, and increased body hair growth (hirsutism). Other common side effects of anabolic steroid use in women include menstrual irregularities, acne, and mood changes.

167. (A) I and II.

Blood doping refers to the practice of artificially enhancing athletic performance by increasing the oxygen-carrying capacity of the blood, which can be achieved by infusing red blood cells or taking erythropoietin (EPO) to increase red blood cell production. Injecting steroids to increase muscle mass and strength is not used in blood doping.

168. (A) Events that require high levels of endurance.

Insulin promotes glucose uptake into the muscle and aids in the formation and storage of glycogen in the muscle. Athletes use insulin for events that require high levels of endurance.

169. (B) Increasing the weight lifted in each workout while keeping the number of repetitions constant.

Increasing the weight lifted in each workout while keeping the number of repetitions constant is an example of progressive overload. To achieve progressive overload, a person must gradually increase the resistance, duration, or intensity of their exercise.

170. (D) Decreasing the intensity of the exercise.

Increasing the weight lifted, increasing the number of repetitions performed, and decreasing the rest period between sets are all ways to implement progressive overload by increasing the stress on the muscles and forcing them to adapt to new challenges. However, decreasing the intensity of the exercise would not provide an increased demand on the body and would not result in progressive overload. Hence, option D is correct.

171. (A) 1-5 repetitions.

The most appropriate repetition range for developing maximal strength is 1-5 repetitions. Training in the lower repetition range with heavier weights is the most effective way to increase maximal strength by stimulating the nervous system to recruit more muscle fibers, improving muscular coordination, and increasing the size and cross-sectional area of the muscle fibers. Higher repetition ranges are more appropriate for muscular endurance or hypertrophy training.

172. (B) Eccentric phase duration.

The first number in a tempo prescription signifies the eccentric phase duration. It is typically expressed as a series of four numbers, such as "3-0-1-0". The first number represents the duration, in seconds, of the eccentric phase, which is the portion of the movement where the muscle lengthens under tension. The second number represents the duration, in seconds, of any pause or isometric hold at the midpoint of the movement. The third number represents the duration, in seconds, of the concentric phase, which is the portion of the movement where the muscle shortens under tension. So, option B is correct.

173. (A) Bench press followed by pull-ups.

An example of a compound set is a bench press followed by pull-ups. A compound set is a training technique where two exercises are performed in rapid succession without rest between them, targeting different muscle groups. Bench press primarily targets the chest, shoulders, and triceps, while pull-ups primarily target the back and biceps. Performing them together in a compound set creates a high demand for the upper body muscles, making the workout more challenging and increasing the training effect. Squats followed by calf raises are an example of a superset, deadlifts followed by leg curls are an example of a pairing, and bench press followed by bicep curls is an example of an antagonist set.

174. (A) Reducing the weight used during a set to allow for more repetitions.

A drop set is a training technique where an exercise is performed with a heavy weight for a set number of repetitions, then immediately followed by reducing the weight and continuing with the same exercise for more repetitions until failure. Hence, from the options, the best answer is A, "a drop set in resistance training is best defined as reducing the weight used during a set to allow for more repetitions."

175. (B) Muscular hypertrophy.

The drop set technique involves reducing the weight used during a set to allow for more repetitions, which increases the amount of time under tension for the targeted muscles. This technique is commonly used in bodybuilding and hypertrophy-focused training to maximize metabolic stress and stimulate muscle growth. Hence, when training an athlete using the drop set technique, the primary training goal is muscular hypertrophy, so option B is correct.

176. (A) Bench press.

The bench press is an example of a compound exercise. A compound exercise is an exercise that involves multiple muscle groups and joints working together to perform the movement. The bench press involves the chest, shoulders, and triceps, as well as the stabilizing muscles of the core and upper back. In contrast, a leg extension is an isolation exercise that only targets the quadriceps muscles of the legs. A lateral raise primarily targets the deltoid muscles of the shoulders, and triceps kickbacks primarily target the triceps muscles of the arms. Hence, the correct option is option A.

177. (C) Maximal strength.

Compound exercises involve multiple muscle groups and joints working together, allowing for the use of heavier weights and the activation of more muscle fibers, resulting in greater overall strength gains. By engaging multiple muscle groups, the body can generate greater force, leading to maximal strength improvements.

178. (A) Estimating one-rep max.

The Brzycki formula is used for estimating one-rep max. One-rep max (1RM) is the maximum amount of weight that a person can lift for one repetition with proper form.

179. (C) The maximum weight that can be lifted for a given number of repetitions.

In strength training, the RM is a measure of an individual's maximal strength and is typically used to determine training loads for a given exercise. Repetition maximum (RM) is the maximum weight that can be lifted for a given number of repetitions

180. (D) Neutral grip.

A pronated grip is where the palms are facing down, and the knuckles are pointing forwards, such as in a pull-up. A supinated grip is where the palms are facing up, and the knuckles are pointing forwards, such as in a bicep curl. An alternated grip is where one hand is pronated, and the other is supinated, and is commonly used in deadlifts. A neutral grip is where the palms are facing each other, and the knuckles are pointing forwards. Option D is correct.

181. (B) To protect the lower back by increasing intra-abdominal pressure.

When lifting heavy weights, there is a risk of lower back injury due to excessive spinal compression. The main reason for athletes wearing a weight belt during lifting is to protect the lower back by increasing intra-abdominal pressure.

182. (A) The spotter should stand behind the lifter.

Over-the-face exercises are those where the weight is lifted over the head, such as overhead press and bench press. These exercises can be dangerous if the lifter fails to complete the lift and the weight comes down toward their face or neck. A spotter can help prevent injury by standing behind the lifter and assisting them if the weight becomes too heavy or the lifter is unable to complete the lift.

183. (B) Grasping the barbell with a narrow, overhand grip.

The high-bar Olympic squat is a technique used in weightlifting that involves placing the barbell on the upper traps and performing a deep squat, lowering the body until the thighs are parallel to the ground or lower. Grasping the barbell with a narrow, overhand grip is not a correct technique used to perform the high-bar Olympic squat.

184. (A) Above the head with the arms fully extended.

The snatch is an Olympic weightlifting movement that involves lifting a barbell from the ground to overhead in one fluid motion. In the final position of the snatch, the lifter should have a stable, balanced position with the barbell held above the head and the arms fully extended.

185. (A) Explosive power.

Olympic weightlifting focuses on explosive power. Olympic weightlifting is a sport in which two lifts are performed with a barbell loaded with weight plates: the snatch and the clean and jerk. Lifting the barbell from the ground to an overhead position requires explosive power from the lifter's legs, hips, and back. While cardiovascular endurance, muscular endurance, and flexibility are all important for overall fitness and athletic performance, Olympic weightlifting isn't one of them.

186. (A) Olympic weightlifting utilizes weights, while plyometric exercise uses bodyweight.

Olympic weightlifting focuses primarily on lifting heavy weights to develop strength and power. Plyometric exercise is a type of training that uses explosive movements with the body weight as resistance, such as jumping or hopping. While plyometric exercises may sometimes incorporate some additional weights, the focus is on bodyweight exercises that enhance explosive power.

187. (B) 16 - 42 inches.

The recommended height for depth jumps ranges from 16 to 42 inches, with 30 to 32 inches being the norm.

188. (A) Leg press.

Examples of ground-based free exercise include Olympic lifts, squats, and deadlifts. Hence, Option A is correct, as the leg press is not an example of a ground-based free-exercise.

189. (D) All of the options use variable resistance.

All of the options—bench presses, squats, and deadlifts—can use variable resistance. Variable resistance refers to a type of resistance that changes throughout the range of motion of an exercise. This type of resistance is typically achieved by using equipment such as resistance bands, chains, or specialized machines.

190. (C) It increases muscle activation throughout the entire range of motion.

Variable resistance involves changing the resistance throughout the range of motion of an exercise, which can increase muscle activation during the weaker portions of the movement. An advantage of using variable resistance during training is that it increases muscle activation throughout the entire range of motion. In contrast, variable resistance does not necessarily reduce the risk of injury, nor does it make the exercise easier to perform.

191. (A) Bench press.

The bench press is the exercise that is most commonly performed using variable resistance. While exercises like bicep curls, leg presses, and lunges can also benefit from variable resistance, they are less commonly performed using this method compared to bench presses.

192. (B) The clean.

The log lift is a strongman exercise that involves lifting a heavy log off the ground and pressing it overhead. It is similar to the clean exercise in weightlifting, which involves lifting a barbell from the ground to the shoulders, using a triple extension of the ankles, knees, and hips. Option B is correct.

193. (D) Bicep curls.

Strongman training involves various functional movements that mimic real-life tasks, such as lifting, pushing, and carrying heavy objects over long distances. Exercises commonly used in strongman training include the deadlift, squat, overhead press, farmer's walk, log press, yoke carry, and tire flip. Bicep curls are typically not associated with strongman training. Hence, option D is correct.

194. (D) Box jump.

The box jump is not a strongman exercise. The deadlift, tire flip, and farmer's walk are all common strongman exercises that test strength, endurance, and overall fitness. The box jump, on the other hand, is a plyometric exercise that focuses on explosive power and lower body strength.

195. (A) Deadlift.

Deadlifts should be performed last in a resistance training program as they engage multiple muscle groups and require a significant amount of energy. It is recommended to perform isolation exercises like lat pulldowns, triceps curls, and leg extensions earlier in a workout, while compound exercises such as squats or lunges can be performed before isolated exercises like leg extensions.

196. (C) 11,400 pounds.

The training volume for the barbell bench press exercise if you perform 6 sets of 10 reps with 190 pounds is:

6 sets x 10 reps x 190 pounds = 11,400 pounds

197. (B) 165 pounds.

To calculate the appropriate training load for the athlete, multiply their estimated one-rep max by the percentage prescribed in the program.

55% of 300 pounds = (55/100) x 300 pounds = 165 pounds

198. (D) All of the options.

All of the options can contribute to fatigue during high-intensity exercise. Depletion of muscle glycogen, accumulation of lactate in the muscles, and increased core temperature can contribute to fatigue during high-intensity exercise.

199. (B) High-intensity, short-duration exercise.

High-intensity, short-duration exercise is the training method that is most effective at improving resistance to fatigue. It does this by improving muscle function. HIIT involves brief, high-intensity bursts of exercise followed by periods of rest or low-intensity exercise.

200. (D) All of the above.

All of the listed factors—training intensity, training frequency, and recovery time—can influence the magnitude and duration of the supercompensation effect.

201. (C) Construction phase.

In general, the construction phase of designing a new strength and conditioning facility takes the longest time. This phase typically takes 50% of the total project time (12 months) and requires strict adherence to set deadlines.

202. (A) Providing adequate space for emergency responders.

Providing adequate space for emergency responders is an important safety consideration when designing a strength and conditioning facility. Accidents and injuries can happen in any fitness facility, and it is important to be prepared for emergencies.

203. (B) 12-14.

The recommended ceiling height in a strength and conditioning facility is 12-14 feet. This height allows for the use of various equipment, such as cable machines, suspension trainers, and Olympic lifting platforms, without risking damage to the ceiling or limiting the range of motion of clients.

204. (C) Barbells and weights.

The aerobic area in a strength and conditioning facility typically houses cardiovascular exercise equipment such as treadmills, elliptical machines, rowing machines, and stationary bikes. Barbells and weights are typically housed in the strength training area, which may be separate from the aerobic area or incorporated into a larger facility. Therefore, the answer is barbells and weights.

205. (C) Proximate Cause.

Proximate cause is an event linked to an injury that a court determines to be responsible for the injury. Option A, negligence, is a failure to act as a reasonable person, includes duty, breach of duty, proximate cause, and damages. Option B, breach of duty, is a failure to fulfill the responsibility to act with appropriate care. Option D, the assumption of risk, is the acknowledgment of inherent risk in participating and choosing to participate anyway. Option C is the correct option.

206. (A) Pull.

The fundamental movement pattern that involves moving weight away from the body is the pull. Pulling involves moving an object or weight closer to the body by using the upper body muscles such as the biceps, back, and shoulders. On the other hand, pushing involves moving weight away from the body using the upper body muscles such as the chest, triceps, and shoulders. Squatting involves lowering the body by bending at the knees and hips and is used to build lower body strength. Hinging involves bending at the hips while keeping the back straight. The correct answer is A.

207. (A) Elbow flexion.

The primary function of the biceps brachii muscle is elbow flexion. The biceps brachii is a muscle located in the front of the upper arm that crosses the elbow joint and attaches to the radius bone of the forearm. When the biceps brachii contracts, it pulls the forearm up toward the shoulder, which is known as elbow flexion. The biceps also play an important role in supination, which is the outward rotation of the forearm.

208. (D) Resistance training with low reps and heavy weights.

Resistance training with low reps and heavy weights is a common technique for improving power production in the lower body. This type of training is designed to improve muscular strength and power by using heavy weights and low reps, which stimulate the fast-twitch muscle fibers responsible for explosive movements. Option A, resistance training with lower weights and high reps, can improve muscular endurance but may not have the same impact on power production as heavy weight lifting. Isometric training and static stretching are not typically used for power production in the lower body. Isometric training improves muscular endurance but not power, while static stretching improves flexibility and range of motion but not power production.

209. (A) Periodization.

Periodization is a recommended technique for monitoring and adjusting training volume and intensity over time. Periodization involves dividing a training program into distinct phases, each with its own focus on specific training goals and training methods. This allows for systematic changes in training volume and intensity changes over time, which can help prevent overtraining and optimize performance gains.

210. (A) Varied exercise selection.

Varied exercise selection is recommended when designing a resistance training program to prevent plateaus and improve long-term progress. Repeating the same exercises can lead to adaptation and reduced progress over time. Introducing new exercises and changing the stimulus can help prevent plateaus and continue to challenge the muscles in different ways.

211. (B) High-intensity interval training (HIIT).

High-intensity interval training (HIIT) is a common technique for improving endurance in aerobic activities. HIIT involves alternating between short periods of high-intensity exercise and periods of lower-intensity recovery or rest. This type of training has been shown to improve cardiovascular fitness, increase oxygen uptake, and improve overall endurance.

212. (C) Agility and anaerobic activity.

The 300-yard shuttle run is commonly used to assess agility and anaerobic activity. The test consists of running back and forth between two points (25 yards apart) six times, for a total distance of 300 yards. The goal is to complete the test as quickly as possible, which necessitates quick changes of direction, acceleration, and deceleration.

213. (A) Eccentric.

The lowering or muscle lengthening phase during exertion is referred to as eccentric contraction or eccentric phase.

214. (C) Concurrent validity.

The high correlation between a 1 RM bench press and other accepted upper body strength tests demonstrates concurrent validity. Concurrent validity refers to how closely a measure relates to other measures already accepted as valid. In this case, the 1 RM bench press is compared to other accepted tests for measuring upper body strength, and the high correlation between them indicates that the 1 RM bench press has concurrent validity as a measure of upper body strength.

215. (A) Sodium.

During physical activity, the body loses electrolytes through sweating. During sweating, sodium is lost at the highest concentration. When sodium is lost through sweat, it can lead to dehydration, fatigue, and muscle cramps. Potassium is another important electrolyte that is lost through sweat; however, it is generally lost at a lower concentration than sodium. Magnesium and phosphorus are important minerals for muscle and bone health, but they are not lost in significant amounts through sweat during physical activity.

216. (C) Polyunsaturated fats.

Polyunsaturated fats are the best type of triglycerides recommended to include in a diet to reduce the risk of coronary artery disease. Polyunsaturated fats can help lower cholesterol levels and reduce the risk of heart disease. Omega-3 and omega-6 fatty acids, which are types of polyunsaturated fats, are particularly beneficial for heart health. Monounsaturated fats are also considered heart-healthy and can help lower LDL (bad) cholesterol levels, but they are not as effective as polyunsaturated fats.

217. (B) Eccentric.

An eccentric muscle action occurs when a muscle lengthens under tension, such as the lowering phase of a bicep curl. This type of muscle action is also known as a "negative" contraction.

218. (B) 4 sets of 10 reps at 70% 1RM.

A set-rep scheme of 4 sets of 10 reps at 70% 1RM is typically considered most effective for increasing muscle size. This rep range and volume is often referred to as hypertrophy training and is designed to stimulate muscle growth by increasing muscle tension, metabolic stress, and muscle damage. The 4 sets of 10 reps at 70% 1RM scheme allows for sufficient volume to stimulate muscle growth, while also providing enough resistance to create a significant stimulus for the muscles. The other set-rep schemes listed can be effective for other training goals, such as strength or power, but are not as effective for hypertrophy.

219. (C) Those in season.

The question asks about the priority for scheduling training sessions in a strength and conditioning facility. Priority should be given to those in season, as they need to maintain their strength and conditioning levels while competing. Preseason and offseason training is also important, but athletes in season should be given priority. Gender is not relevant in determining training priority.

220. (A). 23,324 J

Force = mass x acceleration

Force = 9.8 m/s^2 x 170 kg = 1,666N

Work = force x distance x number of repetitions

Work = 1,666 N x 2m x 7 = 23,324 Joules

Test 3 Questions

1. Which of the following is true about white blood cells?

A. The number of white blood cells increases at rest

B. The white blood cells lack hemoglobin

C. The number of white blood cells decreases during short intensive exercise

D. The white blood cell lacks a nucleus

2. Which of the following transmits impulses from the atrioventricular nodes to the bundle branches?

A. The Purkinje fibers

B. The Bundle of HIS

C. The SA node

D. The AV node

3. Which of the following statements best represents the term "acetylcholine?"

A. A type of neurotransmitter

B. A type of muscle fiber

C. A type of bone cell

D. A type of connective tissue

4. What is the role of the synaptic vesicles in the neuromuscular junction?

A. They contain acetylcholinesterase

B. They are responsible for breaking down acetylcholine

C. They store acetylcholine

D. They contain calcium ions

5. All these are part of the tracheobronchial tree, except?

A. Trachea

B. Pharynx

C. Bronchi

D. Bronchioles

6. Which of the following is not a muscle of the abdominal wall?

A. External abdominal oblique

B. Transversus abdominis

C. Internal abdominal oblique

D. Quadratus lumborum

7. The main inorganic component of the bone is_____?

A. Magnesium silicate

B. Calcium phosphate

C. Magnesium phosphate

D. Calcium silicate

8. All of these are types of cartilages found in the human body, except?

A. Hyaline

B. Elastic

C. Fibrous

D. Osseus

9. Which of the following muscles is non-striated?

A. Smooth muscle

B. Skeletal muscle

C. Cardiac muscle

D. None

10. In what organ does the actual exchange of gas occur?

A. Pleura

B. Alveoli

C. Septa

D. Bronchioles

11. All of these are true about the aerobic energy system, except?

A. The aerobic system is dependent on oxygen

B. It is the fastest way to resynthesize ATP

C. A total of 36 molecules of ATP is made from one molecule of glucose in the process of cellular respiration

D. The aerobic system follows two major pathways: The Krebs cycle and the electron transport chain

12. Which of the following hormones is not fat soluble and thus cannot cross the cell membrane?

A. Cortisol

B. Progesterone

C. Insulin

D. Testosterone

13. What is the appropriate term to describe negative stress?

A. Eustress

B. Distress

C. Overstress

D. Hypostress

14. Which of the following substances has an ergogenic effect and can improve athletic performance by reducing anxiety and tremors during competition?

A. Growth hormone

B. Insulin

C. Beta-blockers

D. Erythropoietin

15. Which of the following cells are responsible for the formation of new bones?

A. Osteoclasts

B. Chondroblasts

C. Osteoblasts

D. Chondrocytes

16. Which of the following nutrients will an athlete utilize most during a game?

A. Proteins

B. Carbohydrates

C. Vitamins

D. Lipids

17. All of the following statements are true, except?

A. The quadriceps femoris muscle straightens the leg at the knee

B. The hamstring muscles flex the knee

C. The gluteal muscles adduct the thigh

D. The iliopsoas muscle straightens the thigh

18. Activities lasting 10 seconds to 2 minutes are mainly supplied by _____.

A. The fast glycolysis system

B. The phosphagen system

C. The oxidative system

D. The triglyceride system

19. _____ is the type of joint found in the skull.

A. Cartilaginous

B. Fibrous

C. Synovial

D. Hyaline

20. What is the term used to describe the process of breaking down glucose to produce ATP in the absence of oxygen?

A. Anaerobic respiration

B. Aerobic respiration

C. Oxidative phosphorylation

D. Photosynthesis

21. The junction between the motor neuron and motor fiber is referred to as _____.

A. Synaptic cleft

B. Neuromuscular junction

C. Interneurons

D. Schwann cells

22. The net ATP produced during aerobic respiration is_____

A. 2

B. 36

C. 38

D. 126

23. Which of the following best defines the term "overload" in the context of strength and conditioning?

A. Training with a load that exceeds the body's ability to recover

B. Performing an excessive number of repetitions in a single set

C. Progressively increasing training demands to promote adaptation

D. Training with weights that are too heavy for proper technique

24. Which of the following is a measure of the amount of blood each ventricle pumps in one minute?

A. Stroke volume

B. Ejection fraction

C. Cardiac output

D. Total peripheral resistance

25. What is the ideal work-rest ratio for a system powered by the phosphagen energy system?

A. 1:3 to 1:5

B. 1:12 to 1:20

C. 1:20 to 1:30

D. 1:1 to 1:3

26. Which of the following is a dome-shaped muscle that plays a major role in respiration?

A. The thorax

B. Mediastinum

C. Diaphragm

D. Pleura cavity

27. Which of the following muscles supports the agonist muscle and helps it to perform the movement more efficiently?

A. Antagonist

B. Stabilizer

C. Prime mover

D. Synergist

28. Which of the following exercises primarily target the hamstrings?

A. Leg curls

B. Leg extensions

C. Calf raises

D. Lunges

29. Which of the following exercises primarily target the triceps?

A. Bicep curls

B. Triceps kickbacks

C. Squats

D. Deadlifts

30. It is recommended that athletes consume what percent of their total daily calories as fat?

A. 10-15%

B. 50-60%

C. 20-35%

D. 35-50%

31. Which of these exercises should a female tennis player avoid when starting a resistance training program to minimize the risk of injury?

A. Performing several variations of an exercise.

B. Using light weight for new exercises.

C. Performing one warm-up set with light weight.

D. Performing basic exercises through a partial range of motion.

32. What would be an appropriate work-to-rest period ratio for interval training to avoid stressing the oxidative energy system?

A. 1:15.

B. 1:10.

C. 1:20.

D. 1:3.

33. When children are compared based on physique maturity or sexual maturation, which of the following ages is used?

A. Biological age

B. Chronological age

C. Training age

D. Developmental age

34. What can understanding the organizational legal and liability issues help a strength and conditioning coach do?

A. Minimize the risk of injury and liability for the organization

B. Develop a program that is consistent with the organization's beliefs and value

C. Ensure the strength and conditioning program adheres to all applicable laws, regulations, and guidelines

D. All of the above

35. What is the recommended ceiling height in a strength and conditioning facility?

A. 16-20 feet

B. 24-32 feet

C. 12-14 feet

D. 8-10 feet

36. What is the goal of periodization in resistance training?

A. To increase the risk of injury by systematically varying the training load and intensity over time

B. To decrease performance by gradually increasing the training volume and intensity over time

C. To optimize performance and reduce the risk of injury by systematically varying the training load and intensity over time

D. To focus on a single fitness component in the training program

37. Which of the following techniques involves gradually exposing an athlete to a fear stimulus in a controlled and safe environment to reduce their anxiety or fear response?

A. Progressive Muscle Relaxation (PMR)

B. Autogenic training

C. Systematic desensitization

D. Guided imagery

38. An athlete is performing 10 repetitions of the snatch exercise at 60% of 1RM. What is the most probable limiting factor?

A. Muscle glycogen and liver glycogen

B. Liver glycogen only

C. Muscle glycogen and fat stores

D. Muscle glycogen and creatine phosphate

39. What is the purpose of the macrocycle in periodization?

A. To organize the daily and weekly training schedule

B. To focus on specific training goals and objectives

C. To plan and organize the overall training program

D. To focus on the final stages of the preparation period

40. Which of the following is not part of the job description of a strength and conditioning specialist?

A. Demonstrating exercises and technique

B. Designing and implementing safe and effective strength and conditioning programs

C. Assessing the physical needs and limitations of athletes and clients

D. Decorating the training facility with artistic elements

41. What muscles are worked in the bench press exercise?

A. Chest, shoulders, and triceps

B. Biceps, back, and abs

C. Glutes, hamstrings, and quads

D. Calves and shins

42. Which equation represents cardiac output?

A. CO= HR × TPR

B. CO= HR − TPR

C. CO= HR × SV

D. CO= HR − SV

43. In which of the following sports would an athlete benefit most from a high concentration of Type II muscle fibers?

A. Long-distance cycling

B. Cross-country skiing

C. Marathon

D. Weight lifting

44. Which of the following is a hormone that stimulates the production of red blood cells and can improve endurance performance?

A. HGH

B. Testosterone

C. EPO

D. Clenbuterol

45. Which exercise is a variation of the deadlift?

A. Lateral raise

B. Sumo deadlift

C. Tricep extension

D. Preacher curl

46. All of these muscles control facial expressions, except _____.

A. Frontalis

B. Buccinator

C. Temporalis muscle

D. Orbicularis oris

47. Long bones are found in the following part of the body except _____.

A. Arms

B. Thighs

C. Forearms

D. Wrist

48. A 32-year-old swimmer is doing a distance workout. Which of the following would not affect her stroke technique?

A. The number of laps she completes

B. Her state of training

C. Her initial motivation levels

D. Her gender

49. In women who are still menstruating, which of the following hormones is at a higher level at rest compared to men?

A. Cortisol

B. Testosterone

C. Growth hormone

D. Insulin

50. Assistance exercises generally target the following muscle groups except _____.

A. The upper arm

B. The thigh

C. The abs

D. The calf

51. Which of the following common supplements used by athletes help with endurance and resistance training?

I. Vitamin E

II. Beta-hydroxy-beta-methylbutyrate (HMB)

III. Betaine

A. I only

B. I and II

C. II and III

D. I and III

52. The act of temporarily lowering the level of intensity, volume, or frequency of a workout to promote recovery and prevent overtraining is referred to as _____.

A. Rest

B. Unloading

C. Recovery

D. De-training

53. What is the main focus of reversal theory in sport and exercise psychology?

A. The relationship between arousal and performance

B. The critical threshold for performance change

C. The role of motivation in behavior and performance

D. The impact of internal states on behavior and performance

54. What type of training program is a collegiate softball player using if she trains her back and biceps on one day and her chest and triceps on the next day?

A. Spilt training

B. Circuit-training

C. Unilateral training

D. Progressive overload

55. What type of resistance training program is most effective for increasing muscular endurance?

A. High load, low repetitions

B. Low load, high repetitions

C. High load, high repetitions

D. Low load, low repetitions

56. The order of exercises is determined by which of the following principles?

A. Principle of maximum reciprocity

B. Principle of fatigue and priority

C. Principle of resistance and recovery

D. Principle of progression and volume

57. An athlete performs 10 repetitions of bicep curls, immediately followed by 10 repetitions of tricep kickbacks. What type of set did she perform?

A. Giant set

B. Super set

C. Drop set

D. Interval set

58. The ideal location for a strength and conditioning facility is on which floor?

A. The ground floor

B. The central floor

C. The topmost floor

D. The second floor

59. Which of the following best describes the "FITT" principle in strength and conditioning?

A. Flexibility, Intensity, Time, and Type

B. Frequency, Intensity, Time, and Type

C. Flexibility, Intensity, Technique, and Time

D. Frequency, Intensity, Technique, and Type

60. What type of grip is an athlete using if they are looking at their palms at the beginning of an exercise?

A. Supinated grip

B. Pronated grip

C. Alternate grip

D. Hook grip

61. Which of the following is generally considered to be the most intense of the following plyometric drills?

A. Multiple hops

B. Jumps in place

C. Box drills

D. Depth jumps

62. Which of the following muscles is primarily responsible for hip extension?

A. Gluteus maximus

B. Hamstrings

C. Quadriceps

D. Iliopsoas

63. One of your athletes has just switched to being a vegetarian; as a result of this diet, she is at risk of being deficient in which of the following?

A. Vitamin A

B. Vitamin B12

C. Vitamin C

D. Vitamin E

64. The ceiling height for standing, box, and depth jumps plyometric exercise facility must be between _____ meters.

A. 10-12

B. 6-8

C. 3-4

D. 1-2

65. According to dietary guidelines, what total fat intake should come from monounsaturated sources?

A. 25%

B. 35%

C. 10%

D. 45%

66. Which surfaces should be avoided during plyometric training of uninjured athletes because they extend the amortization phase?

A. Grass fields

B. Thick exercise mat

C. Rubber mats

D. Suspended floors

67. _____ is the largest vein in the body.

A. Pulmonary vein

B. Vena cava

C. Coronary vein

D. Renal vein

68. During the early support phase of the sprint cycle, which movement helps to minimize the braking effect of the foot strike?

A. Centric torsion

B. Eccentric hip extension

C. Concentric hip extension

D. All of the above

69. You are scheduling a Junior high school football team's use of the strength and conditioning facility. The staff-to-athlete ratio should not exceed _____.

A. 1:10

B. 1:15

C. 1:20

D. 1:25

70. Which of the following is the main aim of a strength and conditioning program?

A. To improve strength and power

B. To improve speed and agility

C. To improve athletic performance

D. To improve flexibility

71. All these are physiological adaptations that occur in response to exercise, except?

A. Increased cardiac output

B. Decreased hemoglobin levels in the blood

C. Muscle hypertrophy

D. Increased myoglobin

72. All these are adaptations in the fast-twitch muscle fibers that lead to the use of anaerobic energy systems, except?

A. Increased anaerobic enzymes for glycolysis

B. Increased creatine phosphate stores

C. Increased capillary density

D. Increased removal of lactate

73. All of the following are adaptations in the slow-twitch muscle fibers that lead to the use of aerobic energy systems, except?

A. Increase of mitochondria

B. Increased capillary density

C. Increased glycogen and fat stores

D. Increased removal of lactate

74. Which of the following is the use of hypnosis in sport and exercise psychology?

A. To increase motivation and performance

B. To decrease anxiety and stress

C. To improve sleep quality

D. All of the above

75. Which of the following is the main difference between the setup for the snatch and the clean and jerk lifts?

A. Hand position on the bar

B. Foot position

C. Grip width on the bar

D. Stance width

76. At what stage of the motor learning process is an athlete beginning to show improvement in performance, with their movements becoming more fluid, reliable, and efficient?

A. Cognitive stage

B. Associative stage

C. Autonomous stage

D. Consolidation stage

77. Which of the following is an indicator of potential mental health issues in athletes?

A. Changes in sleep patterns

B. Withdrawal from social activities

C. Decreased performance

D. All of the above

78. What is the primary role of the hormone insulin during exercise and recovery?

A. Stimulating muscle protein breakdown

B. Mobilizing fatty acids for energy

C. Promoting glucose uptake into muscle cells

D. Stimulating gluconeogenesis

79. What is the primary advantage of using free weights over machines for resistance training?

A. Free weights provide constant resistance

B. Free weights allow for greater exercise variety

C. Free weights isolate specific muscle groups

D. Free weights are less challenging

80. What type of reliability test is used in which multiple raters will score the same test results and then compare the results to see how consistent they are?

A. Inter-rater reliability

B. Test-retest reliability

C. Intra-rater reliability

D. Observer bias

81. What is the primary purpose of the initial needs analysis in designing a strength and conditioning program?

A. To identify an individual's goals and establish a baseline level of fitness

B. To develop an appropriate exercise selection for the individual

C. To determine the appropriate intensity and volume of the program

D. To assess the individual's nutritional status

82. Which of the following goal repetitions, sets, and rest periods most effectively promote muscular hypertrophy?

Goal Repetitions, Sets, Rest period

A. 8, 4, 2 minutes

B. 10, 3, 1 minute 30 seconds

C. 12, 3, 2 minutes

D. 15, 4, 2 minutes 30 seconds

83. Which of the following exercises is an example of a multi-joint or compound exercise?

A. Bicep curl

B. Tricep pushdown

C. Leg extension

D. Lat pulldown

84. Which of the following strength exercises would be executed with high speed and power?

A. Hang clean

B. Deadlift

C. Back barbell squat

D. Bench press

85. Which of the following tests would be the most appropriate for assessing a female field hockey player's speed?

A. 1 RM back squat

B. Pro agility test

C. Cooper test

D. Standing broad jump

86. Which of the following principles is most closely related to progressive overload in resistance training?

A. Specificity

B. Variation

C. Periodization

D. Recovery

87. Which of the following is an example of an exercise that could be performed at the end of a resistance training workout?

A. Barbell squat

B. Bench press

C. Bicep curl

D. Deadlift

88. What happens if an individual violates the facility's rules for the second time?

A. Dismissal from the facility for one day

B. Dismissal from the facility for one week

C. A verbal warning by a staff member

D. Permanent dismissal from the facility

89. Which of the following muscles is primarily responsible for hip extension?

A. Gluteus maximus

B. Quadriceps femoris

C. Gastrocnemius

D. Rectus abdominis

90. A female athlete wants to improve her endurance performance. She currently consumes 2000 kilocalories per day, consisting of 30% fat, 20% protein, and 50% carbohydrate. Which of the following guidelines will be most important to achieve her goal?

A. Decrease carbohydrate, increase protein and fat

B. Increase carbohydrate, decrease protein and fat

C. Maintain current proportions but increase overall calorie intake

D. Decrease overall calorie intake, increase protein and carbohydrate

91. Which of the following are benefits of core training?

I. Improves posture and spinal stability

II. Enhances athletic performance

III. Helps prevent lower back pain

IV. Increases flexibility in the hips and lower back

A. I and II only

B. II and III only

C. I, II, and III only

D. I, III, and IV only

92. The discipline system in place involves a tiered penalty system. After how many offenses will the athlete be dismissed for the rest of the year?

A. 2nd

B. 3rd

C. 4th

D. 5th

93. Which of the following variables is not included in Cunningham's equation for RMR?

A. Age

B. Gender

C. Body weight

D. Height

94. Which of the following physiological adaptations helps athletes maintain high intensities of exercise for longer periods of time?

A. Increased stroke volume and cardiac output

B. Decreased stroke volume and cardiac output

C. Decreased oxygen uptake

D. Decreased hemoglobin level

95. What is the difference between chronological age and somatic age?

A. Chronological age is based on physical maturity, while somatic age is based on the number of years that have passed

B. Chronological age is a measure of overall growth, while somatic age is based on specific body part development

C. Chronological age is a measure of maturity, while somatic age is based on physical activity levels

D. There is no difference between the two

96. Which of the following exercises would be most appropriate for targeting the vastus medialis muscle?

A. Full squat

B. Leg press

C. Terminal knee extension

D. Leg curl

97. Which of the following best describes the principle of specificity in strength and conditioning?

A. Training adaptations are specific to the type of exercise performed

B. The body can only adapt to a single training stimulus at a time

C. The body will adapt specifically to the demands placed on it

D. The body requires a variety of exercises to promote adaptation

98. Which of the following is a common error when performing the bench press?

A. Arching the back excessively during the lift

B. Keeping the elbows close to the body

C. Not fully extending the arms at the top of the movement

D. Lifting the head off the bench during the exercise

99. Which of the following is not a risk factor for cardiovascular disease?

A. Smoking

B. High blood pressure

C. Physical activity

D. High cholesterol

100. What is the term for the contraction of the heart muscle?

A. Systole

B. Diastole

C. Vasodilation

D. Vasoconstriction

101. Which of the following structures in the cardiac conduction system is responsible for the rapid spread of electrical impulses through the ventricles?

A. Atrioventricular (AV) node

B. Bundle of HIS

C. Purkinje fibers

D. Sinoatrial (SA) node

102. The period of time during the cardiac cycle when the heart is relaxed but not filled with blood is referred to as_____.

A. Systole

B. Diastole

C. Isovolumetric contraction

D. Isovolumetric relaxation

103. What are some risk factors for mental health issues in athletes?

A. Being a team captain

B. Participating in individual sports

C. High levels of stress and pressure

D. All of the options

104. Which of the following is not an indicator of mental health issues in athletes?

A. Withdrawal from friends and family

B. Increased irritability or anger

C. Decreased performance in training or competition

D. Improved sleep and eating patterns

105. Which of the following is a potential risk associated with the use of creatine as a supplement?

A. Increased risk of kidney disease

B. Decreased muscle mass

C. Increased risk of osteoporosis

D. Decreased endurance performance

106. Which of the following is a banned method of performance enhancement?

A. Training at high altitude

B. Wearing compression garments

C. Taking creatine supplements

D. Blood doping

107. Which of the following is an example of manipulating the volume of training to implement progressive overload?

A. Increasing the weight lifted in each workout

B. Increasing the number of sets performed for a given exercise

C. Decreasing the number of repetitions performed

D. Increasing the rest period between sets

108. Which of the following repetition ranges is most appropriate for developing muscular hypertrophy?

A. 1-5 repetitions

B. 6-12 repetitions

C. 15-20 repetitions

D. 20+ repetitions

109. Which of the following is the correct order for a tempo prescription?

A. Eccentric, Isometric, Concentric

B. Isometric, Eccentric, Concentric

C. Concentric, Eccentric, Isometric

D. Eccentric, Concentric, Isometric

110. Which of the following best represents a 10-repetition maximum (10RM)?

A. The maximum weight that can be lifted for 5 repetitions

B. The maximum weight that can be lifted for 10 repetitions

C. The maximum weight that can be lifted for 15 repetitions

D. The maximum weight that can be lifted for 20 repetitions

111. Which of the following is an example of a plyometric exercise that targets the upper body?

A. Medicine ball slam

B. Jump squat

C. Lateral bound

D. Burpee

112. What type of grip is recommended for a spotter when spotting overhead exercises?

A. Pronated grip

B. Supinated grip

C. Hook grip

D. Alternated grip

113. Which strongman exercise involves carrying a heavy object in each hand and walking as far as possible?

A. Farmer's walk

B. Atlas stone carry

C. Kettle bag training

D. Log carry

114. Which of the following supplements has been shown to reduce the perception of fatigue during exercise?

A. Caffeine

B. Creatine

C. Beta-alanine

D. BCAAs (branched-chain amino acids)

115. What type of validity is demonstrated when a new exercise program designed to improve endurance produces better results than a program designed to build muscle mass?

A. Content validity

B. Construct validity

C. Concurrent validity

D. Predictive validity

116. What is the power output if it takes an athlete 45 seconds to lift a 150 kg barbell 2 m for 5 repetitions?

A. 327

B. 427

C. 527

D. 627

117. What is the most effective strategy for a wrestler who needs to drop a weight category and increase the percentage of their body that is composed of lean muscle mass before the start of the season?

A. Design a nutrition program

B. Provide a list of low-fat foods

C. Recommend that the wrestler increase protein intake

D. Refer to the school's nutritionist

118. A 17-year-old female athlete is performing a push-up. Which muscles act as the primary elbow extensor?

A. Triceps brachii

B. Biceps brachii

C. Brachioradialis

D. Pronator teres

119. Which of the following best describes the difference between agonist and antagonist muscles?

A. Agonist muscles are responsible for the primary movement, while antagonist muscles oppose the movement

B. Antagonist muscles are responsible for the primary movement, while agonist muscles oppose the movement

C. Agonist muscles are larger muscles, while antagonist muscles are smaller muscles

D. Antagonist muscles are larger muscles, while agonist muscles are smaller

120. When a college wrestler achieves 50 wins in his career, the coach places the wrestler's name and picture places on the wall of the gym. This is an example of _____.

A. Positive reinforcement

B. Negative reinforcement

C. Negative punishment

D. Positive punishment

121. Which of the following is a primary function of the erector spinae muscles?

A. Lateral flexion of the spine

B. Extension of the spine

C. Flexion of the spine

D. Rotation of the spine.

122. Which of these is not a fundamental movement in maximum-velocity sprinting?

A. Early flight

B. Late flight

C. Early support

D. Mid-support

123. What stage of the sprinting movement consists of the concentric hip extension, eccentric plantarflexion, and concentric knee flexion?

A. Early flight

B. Late flight

C. Early support

D. Mid-support

124. What muscle does the lat pulldown use?

A. Triceps brachii

B. Quadriceps femoris

C. Latissimus dorsi

D. Rectus femoris

125. Which of the following factors has the greatest influence on the type of energy system used for a given exercise?

A. Intensity

B. Frequency

C. Duration

D. Mode

126. When performing 45-degree sit-ups with a partner, where should the force used to return the ball to the partner primarily come from?

A. Triceps

B. Abdominal muscles

C. Latissimus dorsi

D. Iliopsoas

127. When performing a squat, which of the following muscle groups is primarily responsible for extending the knees?

A. Hamstrings

B. Quadriceps

C. Gastrocnemius

D. Gluteus maximus

128. During a push-up, which of the following muscle groups is primarily responsible for extending the elbows?

A. Biceps

B. Triceps

C. Pectoralis major

D. Deltoids

129. Which of the following exercises primarily targets the gastrocnemius muscle?

A. Seated calf raise

B. Standing calf raise

C. Leg curl

D. Leg extension

130. During which of the following exercises would the oxidative energy system be primarily used?

A. High-intensity, short-duration exercise

B. Low-intensity, short-duration exercise

C. Moderate-intensity, long-duration exercise

D. Anaerobic exercise

131. All of the following are push exercises except?

A. Bicep curls

B. Bench press

C. Shoulder press

D. Triceps extension

132. The stretching and warm-up area in a strength and conditioning facility should have at least _____ square feet of open space.

A. 20

B. 25

C. 49

D. 39

133. The walkways within the circuit training area should measure between _____ for comfortable movement.

A. 2-5

B. 3-6

C. 4-7

D. 9-12

134. Which of the following dietary supplements are considered stimulants?

A. Caffeine

B. Beta-blockers

C. Diuretics

D. Corticosteroids

135. Which of the following refers to the degree of consistency or repeatability of a test?

A. Reliability

B. Validity

C. Objectivity

D. Precision

136. Which of the following energy systems is the primary energy system at work when the body is at rest?

A. Phosphagen

B. Glycolysis

C. Oxidative

D. Fats

137. Which of the following is an example of a plyometric exercise?

A. Box jump

B. Deadlift

C. Bench press

D. Pull-up

138. During a power clean, which of the following muscle groups is responsible for initiating the first pull off the ground?

A. Glutes

B. Calves

C. Quads

D. Hamstrings

139. Which of the following is not a primary muscle worked if a female gymnast is training with the barbell deadlift exercise?

A. Quadriceps

B. Glutes

C. Hamstrings

D. Calves

140. The design phase of a strength and conditioning facility may consume _____ of the total project time.

A. 10%

B. 25%

C. 35%

D. 50%

141. Which of the following tests is typically used to measure anaerobic capacity?

A. T-Test

B. (VO2max) Tests

C. Wingate Test

D. 1RM

142. Which of the following tests is typically used to measure muscular strength?

A. T-Test

B. Wingate test

C. (VO2max) tests

D. 1RM

143. _____ validity refers to the perceived accuracy of a test or test item by the athlete and other casual observers.

A. Construct

B. Criterion

C. Face

D. Predictive

144. During the concentric phase of a barbell back squat, which of the following muscles acts as the primary hip extensor?

A. Gluteus maximus

B. Quadriceps femoris

C. Hamstrings

D. Adductor Magnus

145. _____ type of reliability test involves administering two different versions of the same test to the same group of people and then comparing the results.

A. Split-half reliability

B. Inter-rater reliability

C. Retest reliability

D. Alternate-form reliability

146. Which of the following refers to the level of effort or difficulty of a training session or exercise, often expressed as a percentage of an individual's maximal effort?

A. Training frequency

B. Training intensity

C. Training volume

D. Training load

147. Which of the following refers to the number of repetitions performed in a single set of an exercise?

A. Repetition maximum

B. Maximum voluntary contraction

C. Resting heart rate

D. Blood pressure

148. Which of the following refers to the number of sets and reps performed during a training session or exercise?

A. Training volume

B. Training load

C. Training intensity

D. Training frequency

149. The relative humidity in a strength and conditioning facility should not exceed _____.

A. 60%

B. 70%

C. 80%

D. 90%

150. The ratio of high school facilities to students should not exceed _____.

A. 1:15

B. 1:20

C. 1:25

D. 1:30

151. Which of the following best describes overreaching?

A. A short-term increase in performance due to increased training intensity

B. A short-term decrease in performance due to fatigue that resolves within a week

C. A chronic decrease in performance due to injury

D. A chronic increase in performance due to increased training volume

152. How long should an unloading phase be expected to last in a periodized training program?

A. 1-2 weeks

B. 3-4 weeks

C. 5-6 weeks

D. It depends on the athlete's individual needs and goals

153. Which of the following is not a tertiary method of recovery?

A. Cryotherapy

B. Compression

C. Massage

D. Dynamic stretching

154. Which of the following activities requires a short rest period for improvement?

A. Weight lifting

B. Endurance exercises

C. Strength training exercises

D. All of the above

155. Which of the following statements about rest and recovery period is correct?

A. High intensity of exercises for large muscle groups might require less recovery time

B. Muscular endurance rest periods of more than 2-5 minutes

C. Wait at least 8 hours before training the same muscle group again

D. Strength and powerlifting have a rest time of about 2-5 mins

156. How does the Golgi tendon organ (GTO) respond to increased tension in a muscle?

A. By causing the muscle to contract more forcefully

B. By inhibiting the muscle's ability to contract

C. By increasing muscle spindle activity

D. By stimulating muscle growth

157. The intensity of an exercise is determined by which of the following?

A. Weight used

B. Number of repetitions

C. Sets

D. All of the above

158. If the primary goal of an athlete is to develop maximum strength, which exercise should come first?

A. Power clean

B. Bench press

C. Squat

D. Leg press

159. A weightlifter is training for maximum power output in the clean and jerk. Which exercise should come first in their training session?

A. Deadlift

B. Clean and jerk

C. Squat

D. Box jump

160. Which of the following is not a muscle of the abdominal wall?

A. Pyramidalis

B. Transversus abdominis

C. Rectus abdominis

D. Pectoralis major

161. Which of the following muscles is the deepest flat muscle?

A. Transversus abdominis

B. Internal abdominal oblique

C. Rectus abdominis

D. Intercostal muscles

162. All these muscles are found on the back except _____.

A. Iliocostalis

B. Trapezius

C. Serratus anterior

D. Longissimus

163. _____ are rod-like organelles that contain sarcomeres.

A. Sarcoplasmic reticulum

B. Myosin

C. Myofibrils

D. Schwann cells

164. _____ helps to cushion and facilitate joint movement, absorb shocks, and lubricate joints.

A. Tendons

B. Cartilage

C. Connective tissue

D. Ligament

165. _____ plane separates the body into front and back parts.

A. Sagittal plane

B. Frontal

C. Transverse

D. Longitudinal

166. _____ are two large tubes that carry air from the trachea into the lung.

A. Bronchioles

B. Bronchi

C. Pleural membrane

D. The thorax

167. Which of the following is the main function of the pleura membrane?

A. To slow the full expansion and contraction of the lungs during breathing

B. Houses the heart and other important structures

C. Allows air to pass in and out of the lungs during respiration

D. Carry air from the windpipe into the lungs

168. Which of the following conduction systems slightly delay electrical impulses, so the atria contracts first, before the ventricles?

A. Ventricles

B. SA node

C. AV node

D. Bundles of HIS

169. What is the estimated age-predicted maximum heart rate of a 35-year-old female who is 6'1" tall and weighs 140 lbs. with a resting heart rate of 60 beats per minute?

A. 150

B. 165

C. 175

D. 185

170. In which phase of the periodization cycle would an athlete most likely focus on developing muscular hypertrophy?

A. Hypertrophy phase

B. Strength phase

C. Power phase

D. Recovery phase

171. _____ age represents the extent of growth in overall height or specific parts of the body, such as limb length.

A. Chronological age

B. Biological age

C. Training age

D. Somatic age

172. The processing of internal and external cues that come to awareness is referred to as _____.

A. Motivation

B. Attention

C. Arousal

D. Skill

173. Which of the following breathing techniques is most appropriate during the concentric phase of a resistance exercise?

A. Inhale

B. Exhale

C. Hold breath

D. Slow, controlled breathing

174. As a general guideline, it is recommended that athletes consume approximately _____ grams of carbohydrates per hour before exercise.

A. 5-15

B. 30-60

C. 60-120

D. More than 120

175. An imbalance of electrolytes in the body may lead to which of the following?

A. Dehydration

B. Cramping

C. Confusion

D. All of the above

176. All of the following are stimulants used in long-duration exercises that necessitate short bursts of energy, except _____.

A. Caffeine

B. Ephedrine

C. Cocaine

D. Creatine

177. Which of the following best describes the "two-for-two" rule for adjusting the load in resistance training?

A. Increase the load if an individual can perform two additional repetitions for two consecutive workouts

B. Decrease the load if an individual cannot perform the desired number of repetitions for two consecutive workouts

C. Increase the load if an individual can perform the desired number of repetitions for two consecutive workouts

D. Both A) and B)

178. Which of the following is the principal source of energy for a muscular contraction?

A. ATP

B. Oxygen

C. NADH

D. Lactic acid

179. Which of the following hormones has the most significant influence on neural changes?

A. Cortisol

B. Growth hormone

C. Testosterone

D. Insulin

180. At rest, which of the following hormones has higher levels in women compared to men?

A. Insulin

B. Cortisol

C. Testosterone

D. Growth hormone

181. Which of the following is a potential side effect of anabolic steroid use in men?

A. Breast enlargement

B. Deepened voice

C. Increased body hair

D. Testicular atrophy

182. What is the recommended rest period between sets during a high-intensity interval training (HIIT) workout?

A. 10 seconds

B. 30 seconds

C. 2 minutes

D. 3 minutes

183. The snatch consists of _____ fundamental components executed as a single fluid lift.

A. 2

B. 3

C. 4

D. 5

184. Which of the following is a reason why athletes weighing over 220 pounds may be more susceptible to injury during plyometric exercises?

A. Increased compressive force on joints.

B. They have higher vertical jump ability

C. They have less joint stability

D. They have a slower reaction time

185. Which of the following combinations best describes a person's physiological response to acute stress?

A. Decreased heart rate and blood pressure

B. Increased heart rate and blood pressure

C. Decreased respiration rate and blood sugar

D. Increased digestion and immune function

186. What is the difference between eustress and distress?

A. Eustress is a positive feeling of stress, while distress is a negative feeling of stress

B. Eustress and distress are the same thing

C. Eustress and distress refer to different physiological responses to stress

D. Eustress is a temporary feeling of anxiety, while distress is a long-lasting feeling of anxiety

187. All these are common errors in sprinting technique, except _____.

A. Hips being too high at the start of the crouch position

B. Stepping out laterally during the initial drive phase

C. Jumping the first stride or stepping over the knee of the stance leg

D. None of the options

188. An 18-year Olympic swimmer attempting a personal record ignores the audience to concentrate solely on her performance. Which of the following abilities is this athlete most likely using to perform the exercise?

A. Selective attention

B. Somatic anxiety

C. Successive approximation

D. Dissociation

189. Which of these is incorrect about the general basics of selecting exercise?

A. Start with the basics such as squats, lunges, and push-ups

B. Start with multi-joint exercises before single joint exercises

C. Prioritize isolation exercises over compound exercises

D. Prioritize exercises that target the rehabilitation of the injured muscle

190. A strength and conditioning coach is analyzing the results of a 10-yard sprint test for a group of football players. Which of the following measures of central tendency would best describe the typical time taken to complete the sprint?

A. Median

B. Average

C. Variance

D. Standard variance

191. When compiling the results of the testing for the 400-meter relay team sprint, the strength and conditioning professional notices that most of the scores are comparable, but there are five scores that are significantly higher than the rest of the scores. In regard to this group, which of the following measures of central tendency is considered to be the most appropriate?

A. Average

B. Median

C. Standard deviation

D. All of the above

192. Which of the following is a type of kettlebell?

A. Cast kettlebell

B. Dumbbell kettlebell

C. Curl kettlebell

D. Farmer's kettlebell

193. In tempo training, what does the fourth digit in the tempo digit represent?

A. The eccentric phase of the exercise

B. Time, if any, to pause between the eccentric and concentric portions of the exercise

C. Time for the concentric phase of the exercise

D. Time, if any, to pause between the concentric and eccentric portions of the exercise

194. The sumo lift is characterized by which of the following?

A. A wide stance with the feet pointed straight ahead

B. A narrow stance with the feet pointed outward

C. A wide stance with the feet pointed outward

D. A narrow stance with the feet pointed straight ahead

195. What is the proper starting position for a conventional deadlift?

A. Bent over at the waist with the knees straight

B. Standing upright with the feet shoulder-width apart

C. Bent over at the waist with the knees slightly bent

D. Standing upright with the feet together

196. Which of the following techniques can be used to prevent rounding of the back during the deadlift exercise?

A. Arching the back excessively

B. Keeping the hips high

C. Maintaining a neutral spine

D. Lifting with the arms

197. Which of the following is a common technique error during the high-bar Olympic squat?

A. Failing to reach parallel

B. Arching the back excessively

C. Letting the knees cave in

D. Lifting with the arms

198. Which of the following is a variation of the barbell back squat?

A. Leg press

B. Bulgarian split squat

C. Romanian deadlift

D. Standing calf raise

199. Which of the following exercises is commonly used to target the adductor muscles?

A. Lateral lunge

B. Barbell hip thrust

C. Split squat

D. Romanian deadlift

200. Which of the following exercises is a compound exercise that targets multiple muscle groups, including the chest, shoulders, and triceps?

A. Barbell bicep curl

B. Standing overhead press

C. Seated tricep extension

D. Dumbbell lateral raise

201. All these are factors that affect exercise techniques, except _____.

A. Differences in body type

B. Muscular strength

C. Power output

D. None of the options

202. All these are psychological factors that affect athlete performance, except _____.

A. Increased aggressiveness and sexual appetite

B. Depression

C. Male pattern baldness

D. Anger

203. Which of these depicts the effect of alcohol on athlete performances?

A. Impaired motor skills

B. Decreased coordination.

C. Impaired balance

D. All of the options

204. Which of the following factors primarily determines an individual's basal metabolic rate (BMR)?

A. Age

B. Gender

C. Body composition

D. Activity level

205. Which of the following are the effects of iron on exercise?

I. Increases oxygen uptake

II. Lowers heart rate

III. Lowers lactate concentrations during exercise.

A. I only

B. I and II

C. II and III

D. I, II, and III

206. Which of the following popular bodybuilding supplements increases hydration?

A. Creatine

B. Caffeine

C. Casein

D. Betaine

207. Which of the following exercises primarily targets the posterior deltoid?

A. Lateral raise

B. Front raise

C. Rear deltoid fly

D. Upright row

208. During exercise, which of the following hormones maintain electrolyte and water homeostasis?

I. The antidiuretic hormone (ADH)

II. The renin-angiotensin-aldosterone system

III. The growth hormone

A. I only

B. I and II

C. II and III

D. I, II, and III

209. _____ is a condition where a person regurgitates partially digested food and either re-chews, re-swallows, or discards it.

A. Pica

B. Rumination disorder

C. Restrictive Food Intake Disorder

D. Bulimia Nervosa

210. Which of the following is a water-soluble vitamin?

A. Vitamin A

B. Vitamin E

C. Vitamin K

D. Vitamin B

211. Which of the following is not true about fats?

A. Fat is the primary fuel source for light to moderate-intensity exercise

B. It provides the quick bursts of energy required for speed

C. 10% of fat intake comes from monounsaturated sources

D. Athletes should consume 20-35% of their total daily calories as fat

212. Which of the following is a simple carbohydrate?

A. Whole grain bread

B. Rice

C. Bagel

D. Jellies

213. _____ is a level assumed to ensure nutritional adequacy when evidence is insufficient to develop an RDA.

A. Recommended Dietary Allowance

B. Tolerable Upper Intake Level (TUL)

C. The Estimated Average Requirement (EAR)

D. Adequate Intake (AI)

214. One arm of an athlete is pulled across the chest and held in position with the other arm. Which muscles are affected by the stretch?

A. Biceps brachii and deltoid

B. Pectoralis major and deltoid

C. Triceps brachii and rhomboids

D. Latissimus dorsi and teres major

215. Which of the following equipment would you recommend to an athlete as the most appropriate for performing the bench press and forward step lunge exercises?

A. Resistance bands and stability balls

B. Barbells and dumbbells

C. Kettlebells and medicine balls

D. Plyometric boxes and agility ladders

216. In which of the following exercises is using a spotter recommended?

A. Bodyweight exercises

B. Stretching

C. Overhead stretches

D. Weightlifting

217. When an athlete pulls weight from the floor in a deadlift, where should the shoulders be in relation to the bar?

A. Behind the bar

B. In front of the bar

C. Directly above the bar

D. It doesn't matter

218. In the exercise known as the lat pull-down, which grip would you suggest a weightlifter use in order to reduce the amount of assistance provided by the biceps brachii muscle?

A. Pronated grip

B. Supinated grip

C. Neutral grip

D. Alternating grip

219. When spotting someone for a dumbbell shoulder press or bench press where should the spotter's hands be?

A. On the lifter's shoulders

B. On the lifter's elbows

C. On the lifter's wrists

D. On the dumbbells

220. Which of the following performance-enhancing drugs is not currently classified as a controlled substance and can be purchased as a legal dietary supplement?

A. Creatine

B. Cocaine

C. Ephedrine

D. Erythropoietin

Test 3 Answers and Explanations

1. (B) The white blood cells lack hemoglobin.

Unlike red blood cells, which contain hemoglobin and are involved in oxygen transport, white blood cells (WBC) do not contain hemoglobin. The number of white blood cells increases during intense exercise and does not decrease. However, the number of white blood cells typically increases during times of infection or inflammation, not at rest. The WBC also contains a nucleus.

2. (B) The Bundle of HIS.

The Bundle of HIS transmits impulses from the atrioventricular (AV) node to the bundle branches. The AV node acts as a gatekeeper slowing down the electrical signal before it reaches the Bundle of HIS. The Bundle of HIS then splits into left and right bundle branches, which deliver the electrical signal to the Purkinje fibers. The Purkinje fibers distribute the signal throughout the ventricles, causing them to contract and pump blood out of the heart. The SA node is responsible for initiating the electrical signal that starts each heartbeat.

3. (A) A type of neurotransmitter.

Acetylcholine is a type of neurotransmitter that is released at nerve endings in many parts of the body, including the brain, spinal cord, and neuromuscular junctions.

4. (C) They store acetylcholine.

The role of synaptic vesicles in the Neuromuscular Junction is to store acetylcholine. When a nerve impulse reaches the end of the neuron, voltage-gated calcium channels open up, and calcium ions flow into the neuron terminal. This influx of calcium ions causes the synaptic vesicles to bind to the presynaptic membrane and release acetylcholine into the synaptic cleft, which is the space between the neuron terminal and the muscle fiber. Therefore, the correct statement from the options is "They store acetylcholine."

5. (B) Pharynx.

The Pharynx is not a part of the tracheobronchial tree. The tracheobronchial tree consists of the trachea, bronchi, bronchioles, and lungs. The pharynx, on the other hand, is part of the respiratory and digestive systems. The pharynx connects the nasal cavity and mouth to the esophagus and larynx.

6. (D) Quadratus lumborum.

The Quadratus lumborum is not a muscle of the abdominal wall. The quadratus lumborum muscle is located in the lower back region and is involved in movements of the trunk and pelvis. The other three muscles listed—the external abdominal oblique, the transversus abdominis, and the internal abdominal oblique—are all muscles of the abdominal wall.

7. (B) Calcium phosphate.

The main inorganic component of the bone is Calcium phosphate. Calcium phosphate makes up about 65% of the total weight of bone tissue. It is in the form of hydroxyapatite crystals, which are responsible for the bone's hardness and ability to resist compression.

8. (D) Osseus.

Osseus is not a type of cartilage found in the human body. "Osseus" refers to bone tissue, which is a different type of connective tissue. The other three options - hyaline, elastic, and fibrous - are types of cartilage found in the body.

9. (A) Smooth muscle.

Smooth muscle is the non-striated muscle. Smooth muscle is found in the walls of internal organs such as the digestive tract, blood vessels, and urinary bladder, where it is responsible for involuntary movements. It is called smooth muscle because it lacks the striated appearance of skeletal and cardiac muscle.

10. (B) Alveoli.

The actual exchange of gasses occurs in the alveoli of the lungs. Alveoli are tiny air sacs in the lungs where the exchange of oxygen and carbon dioxide takes place between the air in the lungs and the bloodstream.

11. (B) It is the fastest way to resynthesize ATP.

Option B is incorrect because the aerobic energy system is the slowest of the three energy systems in terms of ATP production, but it has the largest capacity for ATP production. The other statements are true: The aerobic system is dependent on oxygen for the production of ATP; A total of 36 molecules of ATP is made from one molecule of glucose in the process of cellular respiration via the aerobic system; the aerobic system follows two major pathways: The Krebs cycle and the electron transport chain. Hence the correct answer is option B.

12. (C) Insulin.

Insulin is not fat soluble and thus cannot cross the cell membrane. Unlike the other hormones listed (cortisol, progesterone, and testosterone), insulin is a peptide hormone, meaning it is made up of amino acids and is not fat-soluble. Cortisol, progesterone, and testosterone are steroid hormones that are fat soluble and can easily cross the cell membrane to bind with intracellular receptors.

13. (B) Distress.

The appropriate term to describe negative stress is "distress." Distress is a type of stress that is perceived as negative, harmful, or unpleasant. It is the opposite of eustress, which is a type of stress that is perceived as positive, motivating, or beneficial. Hypostress and overstress are not terms used to describe stress.

14. (C) Beta-blockers.

Beta-blockers have an ergogenic effect and can improve athletic performance by reducing anxiety and tremors during competition. Beta-blockers are a class of drugs that are commonly used to treat high blood pressure, but they are also used in sports to reduce anxiety and tremors that may negatively impact performance.

15. (C) Osteoblasts.

Osteoblasts are responsible for the formation of new bones. Osteoblasts are bone-forming cells that synthesize and secrete the organic matrix of bone tissue, which includes collagen and other proteins.

16. (B) Carbohydrates.

An athlete will utilize carbohydrates the most during a game. Carbohydrates are the primary source of energy for high-intensity exercise and are stored in the muscles and liver as glycogen. During exercise, the body breaks down glycogen into glucose to provide fuel for the muscles. Proteins and lipids can also be used for energy, but they are not as efficient as carbohydrates and are typically only used when glycogen stores are depleted. Vitamins are not a significant source of energy for the body.

17. (D) The iliopsoas muscle straightens the thigh.

The iliopsoas muscle does not straighten the thigh. They are responsible for flexing the thigh at the hip joint. The quadriceps femoris muscle is responsible for extending (straightening) the leg at the knee joint, while the hamstring muscles are responsible for flexing the knee joint. The gluteal muscles are a group of muscles that include the gluteus maximus, medius, and minimus. They are responsible for various actions at the hip joint, including abduction, adduction, and extension. The correct answer is D, as the question specifies "except."

18. (A) The fast glycolysis system.

Activities lasting 10 seconds to 2 minutes are mainly supplied by the fast glycolysis system. This system is also known as the anaerobic glycolysis system, which uses glucose as the fuel source to produce ATP without the need for oxygen. This system can provide energy for activities that require high-intensity efforts lasting between 10 seconds to 2 minutes, such as a 400m sprint or a set of heavy weightlifting.

19. (B) Fibrous.

The type of joint found in the skull is a fibrous joint. Fibrous joints are immovable joints consisting of dense connective tissue, which tightly binds bones together. In the skull, the fibrous joints are called sutures, which are thin layers of fibrous tissue that join the bones of the skull together.

20. (A) Anaerobic respiration.

The term used to describe the process of breaking down glucose to produce ATP in the absence of oxygen is anaerobic respiration. Anaerobic respiration is a metabolic process that occurs in the absence of oxygen and involves the breakdown of glucose (or other organic molecules) to produce ATP and other metabolic byproducts, such as lactate.

21. (B) Neuromuscular junction.

The junction between the motor neuron and motor fiber is referred to as the Neuromuscular junction.

22. (B) 36.

The net ATP molecules obtained from one molecule of glucose during aerobic respiration is 36 (2 from glycolysis, 2 from the Krebs cycle, and 32 from the electron transport chain).

23. (C) Progressively increasing training demands to promote adaptation.

The principle of overload involves progressively increasing the demands placed on the body during training to promote adaptation and improvement in strength, power, endurance, or other fitness components.

24. (C). Cardiac output

Cardiac output (CO) measures the amount of blood each ventricle pumps in one minute. To calculate cardiac output stroke volume (SV) is multiplied by heart rate (HR).

25. (B) 1:12 to 1:20.

The ideal work-to-rest ratio for the phosphagen system is 1:12 to 1:20. To allow for sufficient recovery and replenishment of the Phosphagen system, a work-to-rest ratio of 1:12 to 1:20 is generally recommended. This means that for every 1 second of high-intensity exercise, there should be 12 to 20 seconds of rest or low-intensity activity to allow for adequate recovery before the next bout of high-intensity exercise.

26. (C) Diaphragm.

The diaphragm is a large, dome-shaped muscle separating the chest and abdominal cavity. It is the primary muscle responsible for respiration, as it contracts and relaxes during inhalation and exhalation.

27. (D) Synergist.

The synergist muscle works together with the agonist's muscle to produce a movement. While the agonist muscle is primarily responsible for generating the force necessary to perform the movement, the synergist muscle supports the agonist muscle in its action. The antagonist muscle is the muscle that opposes the action of the agonist muscle and works to slow down or stop the movement. The stabilizer muscle works to stabilize the joint by holding it in place. The prime mover, also known as the agonist, is the muscle primarily responsible for performing the movement.

28. (A) Leg curls.

The exercise that primarily targets the hamstrings is leg curls. Leg curls involve bending the knee against resistance while lying face down on a leg curl machine or using ankle weights or resistance bands to target the hamstring muscles. Leg extensions target the quadriceps muscles in the front of the thigh. Calf raises target the calf muscles in the lower leg. Lunges target several muscles, including the quadriceps, glutes, and hamstrings. However, they are not considered a primary exercise for hamstring isolation. So the best option is A.

29. (B) Tricep kickbacks.

The exercise that primarily targets the triceps is tricep kickbacks. Bicep curls target the bicep muscles in the front of the upper arm. Squats primarily target the quadriceps muscles in the front of the thigh, the glutes, hamstrings, and other leg muscles. Deadlifts target several muscles and are not considered a primary exercise for tricep isolation.

30. (C) 20-35%.

It is generally recommended that athletes consume 20-35% of their total daily calories as fat

31. (D) Performing basic exercises through a partial range of motion.

A female tennis player should avoid performing basic exercises through a partial range of motion when starting a resistance training program to minimize the risk of injury. Partial range of motion exercises can put unnecessary stress on the joints and muscles unnecessarily, leading to potential injuries. Other options are good practices to minimize the risk of injury when starting a resistance training program.

32. (D) 1:3.

To avoid stressing the oxidative energy system during interval training, an appropriate work-to-rest period ratio should be between 1:1 to 1:3. Hence option D is correct.

33. (A) Biological age.

Biological age is a measure of maturity determined by factors such as bone development, physical maturity, and sexual maturity. Hence option A is correct.

34. (D) All of the options.

All of the options are correct. Understanding organizational legal and liability issues can help a strength and conditioning coach minimize the risk of injury and liability for the organization, develop a program that is consistent with the organization's beliefs and values, and ensure the strength and conditioning program adheres to all applicable laws, regulations, and guidelines.

35. (C) 12-14 feet.

A recommended ceiling height is 12-14 feet. This would allow for jumping and explosive activities, including the athlete's height and additional space for exercises such as box jumps, vertical jumps, and Olympic lifting.

36. (C) To optimize performance and reduce the risk of injury by systematically varying the training load and intensity over time.

The purpose of periodization is to systematically vary the training load and intensity to allow for recovery and adaptation, and to prevent overtraining and injury. By adjusting the training volume, intensity, and frequency over time, the athlete can optimize their performance and achieve their goals while minimizing the risk of injury and burnout. Hence option C is correct.

37. (C) Systematic Desensitization.

The technique that involves gradually exposing an athlete to a fear stimulus in a controlled and safe environment to reduce their anxiety or fear response is called Systematic Desensitization. It is often used in sports psychology to help athletes overcome fear, anxiety, and other negative emotions related to their sport or performance.

38. (D) Muscle glycogen and creatine phosphate.

The most probable limiting factor for an athlete performing 10 repetitions of the snatch exercise at 60% of 1RM is likely to be muscle glycogen and creatine phosphate. While liver glycogen and fat stores can also contribute to energy production during exercise, they are not the primary fuel sources for high-intensity exercise such as the snatch exercise.

39. (C) To plan and organize the overall training program.

The purpose of the macrocycle in periodization is to plan and organize the overall training program. The macrocycle is the largest of these time periods, typically lasting six months to a year or more, and it provides the overall structure and framework for the entire training program.

40. (D) Decorating the training facility with artistic elements.

Decorating the training facility with artistic elements is not part of the job description of a strength and conditioning specialist. The primary role of a strength and conditioning specialist is to design and implement safe and effective strength and conditioning programs to help athletes and clients improve their physical performance, prevent injuries, and achieve their fitness goals.

41. (A) Chest, shoulders, and triceps.

The bench press exercise primarily works the chest, shoulders, and triceps muscles. The movement primarily targets the pectoralis major muscle in the chest, as well as the anterior deltoids in the shoulders and the triceps brachii in the arms. While other muscles in the body may be engaged to a lesser extent as stabilizers or synergists, such as the biceps, back, and abs, they are not the primary muscles targeted by the exercise.

42. (C) CO= HR × SV.

The equation that represents Cardiac Output is: CO= HR × SV. Cardiac Output (CO) is the amount of blood pumped by the heart in one minute.

43. (D) Weight lifting.

An athlete would benefit most from a high concentration of Type II muscle fibers in Weight lifting. Type II muscle fibers are fast-twitch muscle fibers that generate a lot of force and power but fatigue quickly. This makes them well-suited for high-intensity, short-duration activities such as weight lifting, where explosive power is necessary to move heavy weights quickly.

44. (C) EPO.

The hormone that stimulates the production of red blood cells and can improve endurance performance is EPO (erythropoietin). EPO is a hormone that is produced naturally by the kidneys and stimulates the production of red blood cells in the bone marrow. By increasing the number of red blood cells in the body, EPO can improve the delivery of oxygen to the muscles during exercise, which can enhance endurance performance.

45. (B) Sumo deadlift.

The exercise variation of a deadlift is a Sumo deadlift. The sumo deadlift is a variation of the conventional deadlift in which the lifter assumes a wide stance with their feet pointing outwards at an angle. This variation of the deadlift is named after the sumo wrestler's starting position, which is similar to the starting position of the sumo deadlift. Lateral raise, tricep extension, and preacher curl are all exercises that work different muscle groups and are not variations of the deadlift.

46. (C) Temporalis muscle.

The frontalis, buccinator, and orbicularis oris are all muscles that are involved in facial expression. In contrast, the temporalis muscle is a muscle of mastication (chewing) located on the side of the head, which is responsible for moving the mandible (lower jaw) during chewing. It does not control facial expressions. Hence option C is correct.

47. (D) Wrist.

Long bones are not found in the wrist. Long bones are bones that are longer than they are wide, with a shaft and two ends. They are found in several parts of the body, including the arms, thighs and forearms.

48. (D) Her gender.

A variety of factors, including body position, arm and leg movements, breathing, overall fitness, and strength influence stroke technique in swimming. However, gender is not a factor that directly affects stroke technique in swimming.

49. (A) Cortisol.

In women who are still menstruating, cortisol is at a higher level at rest compared to men. Women typically have higher levels of cortisol than men, both at rest and in response to stress, due in part to the influence of estrogen on the pituitary gland. In contrast, testosterone is typically higher in men than in women, and growth hormone and insulin levels do not differ significantly between the sexes at rest.

50. (C) The abs.

While assistance exercises can target a variety of muscle groups, they generally do not focus on the abs. The abs (rectus abdominis, obliques, and transverse abdominis) are primarily used for stabilizing the trunk during exercises and activities, rather than generating force or movement.

51. (C) II and III.

Beta-hydroxy-beta-methylbutyrate (HMB) and Betaine are common supplements used by athletes that can help with endurance and resistance training. Vitamin E is an antioxidant that can help to protect cells from oxidative stress, but it does not directly impact endurance or resistance training performance.

52. (B) Unloading.

The act of temporarily lowering the level of intensity, volume, or frequency of a workout to promote recovery and prevent overtraining is referred to as "unloading."

53. (A) The relationship between arousal and performance.

The main focus of Reversal Theory in sport and exercise psychology is the impact of internal states on behavior and performance. Reversal Theory suggests that individuals experience a range of emotional states, such as excitement, anxiety, and boredom, and that these states can affect behavior and performance.

54. (A) Split training.

The type of training program that a collegiate softball player is using if she trains her back and biceps on one day and her chest and triceps on the next day is split training. Split training involves dividing the body into different muscle groups and training each group on different days. This allows for greater focus on specific muscle groups and may also help to prevent overtraining.

55. (B) Low load, high repetitions

A resistance training program that emphasizes low loads and high repetitions is most effective for increasing muscular endurance, as it trains the muscles to perform repeated contractions over an extended period.

56. (B) Principle of fatigue and priority.

The order of exercises is determined by the Principle of Fatigue and Priority. This principle involves arranging exercises in a specific order that maximizes performance and reduces the risk of injury.

57. (B) Super set.

The athlete performed a super set. A super set is a strength training technique that involves performing two exercises back-to-back with little or no rest between them. In this case, the athlete performed bicep curls immediately followed by tricep kickbacks. A giant set is a more advanced variation of a super set that involves performing three or more exercises in a row, while a drop set involves performing an exercise to failure, then immediately reducing the weight, and continuing with another set. An interval set is a type of workout that involves alternating periods of high-intensity exercise with periods of rest or lower-intensity exercise. The correct option is B.

58. (A) The ground floor.

In general, the ground floor is often considered the ideal location for a strength and conditioning facility. This is because the ground floor provides easy access for athletes and coaches and allows for large and heavy equipment to be easily loaded and unloaded.

59. (B) Frequency, Intensity, Time, and Type

The FITT principle in strength and conditioning stands for Frequency, Intensity, Time, and Type, which are the four key components to consider when designing a well-rounded exercise program.

60. (B) pronated.

If the athlete is looking at their palms at the beginning of an exercise, they are using a pronated grip. In a pronated grip, the palms are facing downwards, and the fingers are wrapped around the bar or handle with the knuckles facing upwards.

61. (D) Depth jumps.

Depth jumps are generally regarded as the most intense plyometric drill available. Depth jumps are performed by stepping off a box or platform and immediately jumping as high as possible after landing. This drill puts a lot of strain on the lower body muscles and necessitates explosive power and good landing mechanics.

62. (A) Gluteus maximus.

The gluteus maximus is the primary muscle responsible for hip extension, which involves moving the thigh backward from the hip joint. This muscle plays a critical role in movements like running, jumping, and squatting.

63. (B) Vitamin B12.

The athlete is at risk of being deficient in Vitamin B12 as a result of switching to a vegetarian diet. Vitamin B12 is primarily found in animal products such as meat, fish, eggs, and dairy. Vegetarians who avoid or limit these foods may not get enough vitamin B12 in their diet, which can lead to deficiency over time.

64. (C) 3-4.

The ceiling height in a plyometric exercise facility for standing, box, and depth jumps must be between 3-4 meters to allow for safe performance of jumping and other explosive movements.

65. (C) 10%.

According to the dietary guidelines, 10% of total fat intake should come from monounsaturated fatty acids (MUFAs). MUFAs are considered to be a healthy type of fat that can have a positive impact on heart health.

66. (B) Thick exercise mats.

Thick exercise mats and mini-trampolines are not effective for plyometric training of uninjured athletes because they extend the amortization phase.

67. (B) Vena cava.

The vena cava is the largest vein in the body. It is divided into the superior vena cava and inferior vena cava. The superior vena cava brings blood from the upper half of the body, while the inferior vena cava brings blood from the lower half of the body.

68. (C) Concentric hip extension.

During the early support phase of the sprint cycle, the foot makes contact with the ground, which can cause a braking effect if not controlled properly. Concentric hip extension minimizes the braking effect of a foot strike.

69. (A) 1:10.

The staff-to-athlete ratio in junior high strength and conditioning facilities should not exceed 1:10. This allows for adequate supervision and assistance while ensuring that each athlete receives individual attention.

70. (C) To improve athletic performance.

A strength and conditioning program is designed to improve an athlete's physical abilities, such as strength, power, speed, agility, endurance, and flexibility, in order to enhance their overall athletic performance. Hence the correct option is C.

71. (B) Decreased hemoglobin levels in the blood.

Decreased hemoglobin levels in the blood are not a physiological adaptation that occurs in response to exercise. This is because lower levels of hemoglobin would reduce the amount of oxygen that can be transported in the blood and negatively affect performance. Exercise can increase the demand for oxygen in the body, which leads to physiological adaptations such as increased cardiac output and myoglobin. Hence options A and D are true. Muscle hypertrophy is another adaptation that can occur in response to exercise. Hence option C is equally true. Hence the only incorrect statement is B.

72. (C) Increased capillary density.

Increased capillary density is not an adaptation in the slow twitch muscle fibers that leads to the use of anaerobic energy systems. During intense exercise, fast twitch muscle fibers rely primarily on anaerobic Energy systems, such as glycolysis and phosphocreatine, to generate energy. Adaptations that increase the availability and efficiency of these energy systems, such as increased anaerobic enzymes for glycolysis and Creatine phosphate stores, are important for optimal performance. Increased removal of lactate can also delay fatigue during high-intensity exercise. However, increased capillary density is an adaptation in slow twitch muscle fibers that enhances aerobic metabolism and endurance performance, rather than anaerobic metabolism. Hence option C is correct.

73. (D) Increased removal of lactate.

Increased removal of lactate is not an adaptation in slow twitch muscle fibers that leads to the use of aerobic energy systems. Rather, the removal of lactate is an important step in the anaerobic energy system, which is used during high-intensity, short-duration activities such as sprinting and weightlifting.

74. (D) All of the above.

All of the above are potential uses of hypnosis in sport and exercise psychology. Hypnosis can be used to increase motivation and performance by helping athletes to develop positive self-talk, visualization skills, and a sense of self-efficacy.

75. (C) Grip width on the bar.

The main difference between the setup for the snatch and the clean and jerk lifts is the grip width on the bar. In the snatch lift, the grip is wider than in the clean and jerk lift. Specifically, in the snatch lift, the grip is usually placed outside of the knees and the hands are positioned wider than shoulder-width apart, whereas in the clean and jerk lift, the grip is usually placed inside the knees and the hands are positioned closer together, typically about shoulder-width apart.

76. (B) Associative stage.

The stage of motor learning where an athlete begins to show improvement in performance, with their movements becoming more fluid, reliable, and efficient is the associative stage. During this stage, the athlete has already acquired the basic movement pattern and is now refining their movements to make them more consistent and accurate.

77. (D) All of the above.

All of the above are potential indicators of mental health issues in athletes. Changes in sleep patterns, such as difficulty falling asleep, waking up frequently during the night, or sleeping excessively, can be a sign of anxiety, depression, or other mental health concerns.

78. (C) Promoting glucose uptake into muscle cells

Insulin plays a crucial role during exercise and recovery by promoting glucose uptake into muscle cells, which helps maintain blood sugar levels and supports glycogen synthesis for energy storage.

79. (B) Free weights allow for greater exercise variety.

The primary advantage of using free weights over machines for resistance training is that free weights allow for greater exercise variety and more functional, multi-joint movements that better mimic real-life activities.

80. (A) Inter-rater reliability.

The type of reliability test that is used in which multiple raters will score the same test results and then compare the results to see how consistent they are is inter-rater reliability. Inter-rater reliability measures the level of agreement or consistency between different raters or observers who are measuring the same thing.

81. (A) To identify an individual's goals and establish a baseline level of fitness.

The primary purpose of the initial needs analysis in designing a strength and conditioning program is to identify an individual's goals and establish a baseline level of fitness. This information helps guide the development of a personalized program that addresses the individual's specific needs and objectives.

82. (C) 12 repetitions, 3 sets, 2 minutes rest.

According to current research, the best way to promote muscular hypertrophy is to combine moderate to high repetitions (8-12), moderate to high volume (3-5 sets per exercise), and shorter rest periods (60-90 seconds). As a result, option C (12 repetitions, 3 sets, 2 minutes rest) is the most effective for promoting muscular hypertrophy because the repetitions, sets, and rest periods are all within the recommended ranges.

83. (D) Lat pulldown

A multi-joint or compound exercise involves movement at more than one joint and engages multiple muscle groups. The lat pulldown is an example of a compound exercise, as it involves movement at both the shoulder and elbow joints.

84. (A) Hang Clean.

The strength exercise that would be executed with high speed and power is the Hang Clean. The Hang Clean is a multi-joint exercise that involves lifting a barbell in one explosive motion from a hanging position (at thigh level) to a racked position (on the shoulders). To lift the weight quickly and explosively, the lifter must generate a high amount of force and power, making it an ideal exercise for developing power, speed, and explosiveness.

85. (B) Pro Agility Test.

The Pro Agility Test is the best way to assess a female field hockey player's speed. The Pro Agility Test, also known as the 5-10-5 shuttle run, is a popular sport agility and speed test. It entails running 5 yards to one side, then 10 yards the other way, before returning to the starting line for a total distance of 20 yards. The test necessitates quick changes of direction and acceleration, both of which are important aspects of field hockey speed.

86. (C) Periodization.

Periodization is the principle most closely related to progressive overload in resistance training. The use of progressive overload is often incorporated into a periodized program, as the intensity, volume, and/or frequency of the workouts are gradually increased over time to continually challenge the body and promote adaptation.

87. (C) Bicep curl.

Bicep curl is an example of an exercise that could be performed at the end of a resistance training workout. Bicep curls are often included as an accessory exercise at the end of a resistance training workout, after the primary exercises for larger muscle groups (such as squats, deadlifts, or bench presses) have been completed. This allows the biceps muscles to be targeted specifically and can help to increase overall arm strength and size.

88. (A) Dismissal from the facility for one day.

If a second offense occurs, the person will be dismissed from the facility for a day, and the offense will be documented.

89. (A) Gluteus maximus.

The muscle primarily responsible for hip extension is the Gluteus maximus. The gluteus maximus is the primary muscle responsible for hip extension, along with the hamstrings and adductor magnus. In contrast, the quadriceps femoris is a group of four muscles located in the front of the thigh and is responsible for knee extension, not hip extension. The gastrocnemius is a muscle located in the calf that is responsible for ankle plantar flexion, not hip extension. The rectus abdominis is a muscle located in the abdomen that is responsible for trunk flexion, not hip extension. Hence, the correct answer is A.

90. (B) Increase carbohydrate intake, decrease protein and fat.

The most important guideline to improve the endurance performance of a female athlete in this scenario would be to increase carbohydrate intake, decrease protein and fat intake, and maintain current overall calorie intake.

91. (C) I, II, and III only.

The benefits of core training are I, II, and III only. Core training improves posture and spinal stability, enhances athletic performance, and helps prevent lower back pain. However, core training does not typically target the hips and lower back for increasing flexibility. So, the correct answer is I, II, and III only.

92. (C) 4th.

For a fourth offense, the person will be dismissed for the rest of the year, and for the fifth offense, they will be permanently dismissed from the facility.

93. (D) Height.

Cunningham's equation for RMR (resting metabolic rate) includes the variables of age, gender, body weight, and lean body mass. Therefore, height is the variable that is not included in Cunningham's equation for RMR.

94. (A) Increased stroke volume and cardiac output.

Increased stroke volume and cardiac output help athletes maintain high intensities of exercise for longer periods of time. During exercise training, the heart becomes more efficient at pumping blood, which results in an increase in stroke volume and cardiac output. This means that more blood and oxygen can be delivered to the working muscles, allowing athletes to maintain high intensities of exercise for longer periods of time. In contrast, a decreased stroke volume and cardiac output would make it more difficult for athletes to maintain high intensities of exercise for longer periods of time.

95. (C.) Chronological age is based on physical maturity, while somatic age is based on the number of years that have passed.

Chronological age refers to the number of years that have passed since an individual's birth. It is a measure of time that is used to track an individual's overall growth and development. On the other hand, somatic age is a measure of an individual's physical maturity. It is based on specific body part development and can be influenced by factors such as nutrition, physical activity, and environmental conditions.

96. (C) Terminal knee extension.

Terminal knee extension specifically targets the vastus medialis muscle, which is responsible for the last few degrees of knee extension and helps maintain proper patellar tracking.

97. (C) The body will adapt specifically to the demands placed on it.

The principle of specificity emphasizes that the body adapts specifically to the demands placed on it, making it essential to design training programs that target specific goals or desired adaptations.

98. (A) Arching the back excessively during the lift.

One common error when performing the bench press is arching the back excessively during the lift. While some degree of arching in the lower back is necessary to maintain stability during the bench press, excessive arching can put excessive strain on the lower back and increase the risk of injury.

99. (C) Physical activity.

Physical activity is not a risk factor for cardiovascular disease. In fact, physical activity is associated with a lower risk of cardiovascular disease.

100. (A) Systole.

The term for the contraction of the heart muscle is systole. During systole, the ventricles of the heart contract, pushing blood out of the heart and into the arteries.

101. (C) Purkinje fibers.

The structure in the Cardiac Conduction System that is responsible for the rapid spread of electrical impulses through the ventricles is the Purkinje fibers. These fibers are specialized cardiac muscle fibers that conduct electrical impulses rapidly and efficiently throughout the ventricles, allowing for coordinated and synchronized contraction of the ventricular muscle.

102. (D) Isovolumetric relaxation.

The period of time during the Cardiac Cycle when the heart is relaxed but not filling with blood is referred to as "Isovolumetric relaxation." During diastole, the heart is in a state of relaxation and the ventricles are filling with blood from the atria. However, there is a brief period of time within the diastole where the heart is relaxed but not filled with blood. This period is called "isovolumetric relaxation."

103. (D) All of the options.

Being a team captain, participating in individual sports, and high levels of stress and pressure are all risk factors for mental health issues in athletes.

104. (D) Improved sleep and eating patterns.

Improved sleep and eating patterns are not an indicator of mental health issues in athletes. In fact, improved sleep and eating patterns are often signs of good mental health. However, the other options - withdrawal from friends and family, increased irritability or anger, and decreased performance in training or competition - are all potential indicators of mental health issues in athletes.

105. (A) Decreased endurance performance.

One potential risk associated with using creatine as a supplement is an increased risk of kidney disease. Although creatine is generally considered safe and effective for most people when used as directed, excessive use or use by individuals with pre-existing kidney disease may increase the risk of kidney damage. Decreased muscle mass, increased risk of osteoporosis, and decreased endurance performance is not typically associated with creatine use.

106. (D) Blood doping.

Blood doping is a banned method of performance enhancement. Blood doping is artificially increasing the number of red blood cells in the body, which can improve an athlete's endurance and performance. Most sports organizations ban blood doping because it can have serious health consequences, including an increased risk of heart attack, stroke, and blood clots.

107. (B) Increasing the number of sets performed for a given exercise.

The correct answer is increasing the number of sets performed for a given exercise. Manipulating the volume of training is one way to implement progressive overload, and increasing the number of sets performed for a given exercise is an example. Increasing the weight lifted in each workout is an example of progressive overload through increasing intensity, rather than volume. Furthermore, decreasing the number of repetitions performed is also an example of intensity-based overload. Increasing the rest period between sets is a way to modify the training density, but not necessarily the volume of training.

108. (B) 6-12 repetitions.

The repetition range that is most appropriate for developing muscular hypertrophy is 6-12 repetitions. This is because it falls within the "hypertrophy range," which is typically defined as 6-15 repetitions per set.

109. (A) Eccentric, Isometric, Concentric.

The correct order for a tempo prescription is Eccentric, Isometric, and Concentric. This is because tempo prescriptions typically refer to the timing or speed of each phase of a repetition.

110. (B) The maximum amount of weight that can be lifted for 10 reps.

A 10-repetition maximum (10RM) represents the maximum weight that can be lifted for 10 repetitions. This is because 10RM refers to the maximum amount of weight that can be lifted for 10 reps with good form and without reaching failure.

111. (A) Medicine ball slam.

Medicine ball slam is an example of a plyometric exercise that targets the upper body. A medicine ball slam is performed by holding a medicine ball overhead and slamming it into the ground explosively. This exercise works the upper body muscles, such as the shoulders, chest, and triceps, as well as the core and legs, to produce power and stability. The other exercises listed are plyometric exercises for the lower body (jump squat, lateral bound) or a combination of upper and lower body movements (burpee).

112. (A) Pronated grip.

When spotting overhead exercises, a spotter should use a pronated grip. This is a grip where the palms are facing downward, and the fingers are wrapped around the bar or weight from below. This grip allows the spotter to have a secure hold on the weight and provide assistance or take control if necessary, while also allowing the lifter to maintain their grip and control of the weight.

113. (A) Farmer's walk.

The strongman exercise that involves carrying a heavy object in each hand and walking as far as possible is called the Farmer's walk. This exercise involves picking up a weight in each hand, such as a pair of dumbbells or loaded farmer's walk handles, and walking as far as possible without dropping the weights.

114. (C) Beta-alanine.

Beta-alanine has been shown to reduce the perception of fatigue during exercise. Beta-alanine improves exercise performance and delays fatigue during high-intensity exercise by reducing the accumulation of hydrogen ions that contribute to muscle fatigue. Caffeine, creatine, and BCAAs have also been shown to have various benefits for exercise performance, but they do not directly affect the perception of fatigue.

115. (B) Construct validity.

The type of validity demonstrated when a new exercise program designed to improve endurance produces better results than a program designed to build muscle mass is construct validity. Construct validity refers to the degree to which a test or measurement accurately measures the theoretical construct or concept it is intended to measure. For this question, the theoretical constructs being measured are endurance and muscle mass, and the exercise programs are designed to manipulate these constructs. By showing that the endurance program produces better results than the muscle mass program, it demonstrates the construct validity of the program for improving endurance.

116. (A) 327.

Power = Work / Time

Work = Force x Distance

To find the Force, we need to multiply the weight by the acceleration due to gravity (9.81 m/s^2):

Force = Weight x 9.81

Force = 150 kg x 9.81 = 1,471.5 N

The distance lifted is 2 m per repetition, so the total distance lifted for 5 repetitions is:

Distance = 2 m x 5 = 10 m

Then Work = Force x Distance

Work = 1,471.5 N x 10 m = 14,715 J

Finally, we can calculate the Power:

Power = Work / Time

Power = 14,715 J / 45 s = 327 W

Therefore, the power output is 327 W.

117. (A) Design a nutrition program.

The most appropriate course of action for a wrestler who needs to drop a weight category and increase lean muscle mass before the season begins is to design a nutrition program. Dropping a weight category while maintaining or increasing muscle mass requires careful nutrition and exercise planning. Referring to the school's nutritionist can also be helpful in developing a nutrition plan that meets the athlete's needs.

118. (A) Triceps brachii.

The primary elbow extensor muscle during a push-up is the triceps brachii. The triceps brachii is a three-headed muscle located on the posterior side of the upper arm and is responsible for extending the elbow joint. It is heavily used during exercises that require pushing movements, such as push-ups, bench presses, and dips.

119. (A) Agonist muscles are responsible for the primary movement, while antagonist muscles oppose the movement.

Agonist muscles are responsible for producing the primary movement in an exercise, while antagonist muscles oppose or reverse the movement. In many cases, the antagonist muscles work to stabilize the joint and control the speed of movement.

120. (A) Positive reinforcement.

This is an example of positive reinforcement. Positive reinforcement is a process in which a desirable behavior is reinforced or rewarded, increasing the likelihood of that behavior being repeated in the future.

121. (B) Extension of the spine

The primary function of the erector spinae muscles, which include the iliocostalis, longissimus, and spinalis muscles, is to extend the spine. They also play a role in lateral flexion and rotation of the spine.

122. (D) Mid-support.

"Mid-support" is not a fundamental movement in maximum-velocity sprinting. The five fundamental movements in maximum-velocity sprinting are early flight, mid-flight, late flight, early support, and late support.

123. (C) Early Support.

The stage of the sprinting movement that consists of the concentric hip extension, eccentric plantarflexion, and concentric knee flexion is known as Early Support.

124. (C) Latissimus Dorsi.

The Lat Pulldown primarily uses the Latissimus Dorsi muscle, which is a large muscle in the back responsible for shoulder extension, adduction, and internal rotation. It is commonly referred to as the "lats" and is the target muscle group for the Lat Pulldown exercise.

125. (A) Intensity.

Intensity has the greatest influence on the type of energy system used for a given exercise.

126. (B) Abdominal muscles.

When performing 45-degree sit-ups with a partner and returning the ball to the partner, the force used to return the ball should primarily come from the abdominal muscles. The 45-degree sit-up is an exercise that targets the rectus abdominis, which is the muscle responsible for flexing the spine. When returning the ball to the partner, the abdominal muscles must contract concentrically to flex the spine forward and generate the force necessary to throw the ball back to the partner.

127. (B) Quadriceps.

When performing a squat, the quadriceps muscle group is primarily responsible for extending the knees. The quadriceps muscle group is located at the front of the thigh and consists of four muscles: rectus femoris, vastus lateralis, vastus intermedius, and vastus medialis. These muscles work together to extend the knee joint, which is a key movement involved in performing a squat.

128. (B) Triceps.

During a push-up, the triceps muscle group is primarily responsible for extending the elbows. The triceps muscle group is located at the back of the upper arm and consists of three heads: the long head, lateral head, and medial head. These muscles work together to extend the elbow joint, which is a key movement involved in performing a push-up.

129. (B) Standing calf raise.

The standing calf raise primarily targets the gastrocnemius muscle, which is one of the major muscles responsible for plantarflexion of the ankle joint.

130. (C) Moderate-intensity, long-duration exercise.

The oxidative energy system (also known as aerobic energy system) is primarily used during moderate-intensity, long-duration exercise, where oxygen is readily available to the working muscles. The high-intensity, short-duration exercise, and anaerobic exercise primarily rely on the anaerobic energy systems (phosphagen and glycolytic systems) for energy production, which do not require oxygen. Low-intensity, short-duration exercise may depend on both anaerobic and oxidative energy systems, depending on the intensity and duration of the exercise.

131. (A) Bicep curls.

Bench press, shoulder press, and triceps extension are not pull exercises. They are push exercises because they involve pushing a weight away from the body. Bicep curls, on the other hand, are a pull exercise because they involve pulling a weight toward the body using the biceps muscle.

132. (C) 49.

The stretching and warm-up area should have soft tissue instruments, mats, or bands and at least 49 square feet of open space.

133. (C) 4-7.

The walkways within the circuit training area should measure between 4-7 feet (1.2-2.1 m) for comfortable movement.

134. (A) Caffeine.

Caffeine is the only one among the four dietary supplements listed that is considered a stimulant. Beta blockers, diuretics and corticosteroids are not stimulants.

135. (A) Reliability.

The degree of consistency or repeatability of a test is referred to as "reliability."

136. (C) Oxidative.

When the body is at rest, the primary energy system at work is the oxidative system. The oxidative system relies on the aerobic metabolism of carbohydrates, fats, and proteins to produce ATP, which provides energy for the body's ongoing physiological functions

137. (A) Box jump

The box jump is an example of a plyometric exercise, which involves rapid, explosive movements that take advantage of the stretch-shortening cycle to improve power and speed.

138. (C) Quads.

During a power clean, the quadriceps (quads) are primarily responsible for initiating the first pull off the ground. During the first pull, the quadriceps are responsible for extending the knees and lifting the barbell off the ground. The glutes and hamstrings also contribute to the movement by extending the hips, but the quads are the primary initiators of the first pull.

139. (D) Calves.

The primary muscles worked during the barbell deadlift exercise for a female gymnast include the glutes, hamstrings, and quadriceps. The calves also play a role in the exercise but are not considered primary muscles in this work out.

140. (A) 10%.

This phase may consume 10-12% of the total project time (around 3 months), where the coach works with an architect to finalize plans, determine equipment needs, and design the facility for user-friendly access for all athletes.

141. (C) Wingate Test.

The Wingate Test is typically used to measure anaerobic capacity. The Wingate Test is a brief (30-second) maximal cycling test that measures peak power, mean power, and fatigue index. It is designed to specifically target the anaerobic energy system and provides an indication of an individual's ability to sustain high-intensity exercise for short durations.

142. (D) 1RM.

The 1 RM (One Repetition Maximum) is typically used to measure muscular strength. The T-Test is a test used to measure agility and speed in sports performance. The Wingate Test is a test used to measure anaerobic power and capacity. VO2max tests are used to measure cardiovascular endurance and aerobic capacity. The correct answer was D.

143. (C) Face.

Face validity refers to the perceived accuracy of a test or test item by the athlete and other casual observers.

144. (A) Gluteus maximus.

During the concentric phase of a barbell back squat, the primary hip extensor is the gluteus maximus muscle. The gluteus maximus is the largest muscle in the buttocks and is responsible for extending the hip joint. While the quadriceps femoris and hamstrings are involved in the squat movement, they are primarily responsible for knee extension and knee flexion respectively, and the adductor magnus is involved in hip adduction and extension.

145. (D) Alternate-form reliability.

Alternate-form reliability involves administering two different versions of the same test to the same group of people and then comparing the results.

146. (B) Training intensity.

Training intensity refers to the level of effort or difficulty of a training session or exercise, often expressed as a percentage of an individual's maximal effort.

147. (A) Repetition maximum.

Repetition maximum (RM) is a term used in strength training to refer to the maximum number of repetitions a person can perform with a given weight for a particular exercise. The most commonly used RMs are 1RM (one repetition maximum), 5RM (five repetition maximum), and 10RM (ten repetition maximum).

148. (A) Training volume.

Training volume refers to the number of sets and reps performed during a training session or exercise.

149. (A) 60%.

The relative humidity in a strength and conditioning facility should not exceed 60%. This is to help to ensure optimal conditions for exercise, improve comfort and safety, and enhance performance.

150. (A) 1:15.

The ratio of high school facilities to students should not exceed 1:15.

151. (B) A short-term decrease in performance due to fatigue that resolves within a week.

Overreaching is a short-term decrease in performance due to fatigue that resolves within a week. This technique can help to stimulate adaptation and improve athletic performance.

152. (A) 1-2 weeks.

A typical unloading phase, on the other hand, may last between 1-2 weeks. In a periodized training program, the length of an unloading phase is determined by the athlete's individual needs and goals.

153. (D) Dynamic stretching.

Dynamic stretching is not a tertiary method of recovery. It is a type of warm-up or mobility exercise that is typically performed before a workout or competition.

154. (B) Endurance exercises.

Muscular endurance training is a type of strength training that typically involves short rest periods between 20-60 seconds. The goal of this type of training is to increase the ability of the muscles to contract repeatedly over an extended period of time without fatigue.

155. (D) Strength and powerlifting exercises typically require rest periods of about 2-5 min.

Strength and powerlifting exercises typically require rest periods of about 2-5 minutes between sets to allow for the recovery of the muscles and the restoration of energy stores, while muscular endurance training typically involves shorter rest periods of 20-60 seconds to improve cardiovascular fitness and endurance. Option A is wrong because high-intensity exercises for large muscle groups may require more, not less, recovery time to allow for proper recovery and prevent injury. Option C is wrong because it is generally recommended to wait at least 48 hours before training the same muscle group again to allow for full recovery and prevent overuse injuries. Hence the correct option is D.

156. (B) By inhibiting the muscle's ability to contract.

The Golgi tendon organ (GTO) is a proprioceptive sensory receptor found in tendons that responds to increased tension in a muscle. When tension reaches a certain threshold, the GTO inhibits the muscle's ability to contract, which helps prevent injury from excessive force.

157. (D) All of the options.

The intensity of an exercise is determined by a combination of the weight used, number of repetitions, and sets performed. Therefore, all of the options contribute to the intensity of the exercise.

158. (C) Squat.

If the primary goal of an athlete is to develop maximum strength, the squat exercise should come first. The squat is a compound exercise that engages multiple muscle groups, including the legs, hips, and back. It has been shown to be one of the most effective exercises for building lower body strength and power. While the power clean, bench press, and leg press are all important exercises for developing strength, they are typically regarded as secondary to the squat in terms of effectiveness and overall impact on strength development. Hence the correct answer is C.

159. (B) Clean and jerk.

If a weightlifter is training for maximum power output in the clean and jerk, the clean and jerk should be the first exercise in their workout. The clean and jerk is a difficult compound exercise that requires a lot of power, speed, and coordination. When the athlete is fresh, performing the clean and jerk early in the training session can help ensure that they are able to perform the exercise with maximum power and technique.

160. (D) Pectoralis major.

Pectoralis major is not a muscle of the abdominal wall. The pectoralis major is a large muscle of the chest that is responsible for movements of the shoulder joint, such as shoulder flexion, adduction, and internal rotation. It is not a muscle of the abdominal wall. The muscles of the abdominal wall include the rectus abdominis, external oblique, internal oblique, and transversus abdominis, as well as the pyramidalis muscle.

161. (A) Transversus abdominis.

The transversus abdominis is the deepest of the flat muscles of the abdomen. It is located beneath the internal oblique muscle and runs horizontally across the abdomen.

162. (C) Serratus anterior.

Serratus anterior is not a muscle found on the back. The serratus anterior muscle is located on the lateral (side) surface of the rib cage, wrapping around from the front to the back of the torso. The iliocostalis and longissimus muscles are located on either side of the vertebral column in the back. The trapezius muscle is a large, triangular muscle that extends from the base of the skull down to the mid-back and out to the shoulders. Hence the correct answer is Serratus anterior.

163. (C) Myofibrils.

Myofibrils are rod-like organelles made up of repeating units called sarcomeres, which contain the contractile proteins actin and myosin. Hence option C is correct.

164. (B) Cartilage.

Cartilage helps to cushion and facilitate joint movement, absorb shocks, and lubricate joints. Tendons attach muscle to bone and transmit force from muscle to bone. Ligaments attach bone to bone and help to stabilize joints. Connective tissue is a general term that includes tendons, ligaments, cartilage, bone, and adipose tissue. Hence option B is correct.

165. (B) Frontal.

The frontal plane separates the body into front and back parts, while the sagittal plane separates the body into left and right parts, and the transverse plane separates the body into top and bottom parts. The longitudinal plane is not a commonly used anatomical plane. Hence the correct option is B.

166. (B) Bronchi.

The correct answer is "Bronchi." The bronchi are the two large tubes that branch off from the trachea and carry air into the lungs.

167. (A) To slow the full expansion and contraction of the lungs during breathing.

The main function of the pleura membrane is to slow the full expansion and contraction of the lungs during breathing.

168. (C) AV node.

The correct answer is the AV node. The AV (atrioventricular) node is a specialized tissue in the heart that acts as a gatekeeper for electrical impulses traveling from the atria to the ventricles. It slightly delays the impulse, allowing time for the atria to contract and fill the ventricles with blood before the ventricles contract.

169. (D) 185.

The estimated age-predicted maximum heart rate can be calculated using the formula: 220 - age.

So, for a 35-year-old female, the estimated age-predicted maximum heart rate would be 220 - 35 = 185 beats per minute.

170. (A) Hypertrophy phase.

The hypertrophy phase of the periodization cycle focuses on increasing muscle size through moderate-to-high volume training with moderate intensity, typically

171. (D) Somatic age.

Somatic age represents the extent of growth in overall height or specific parts of the body such as limb length.

172. (B) Attention.

The processing of internal and external cues that come to awareness is referred to as Attention. Attention is the cognitive process that allows an individual to selectively focus on specific aspects of their environment while ignoring other distracting stimuli.

173. (B) Exhale.

During the concentric phase of a resistance exercise, it is most appropriate to exhale. This breathing technique helps maintain proper intra-abdominal pressure and prevents excessive increases in blood pressure during exercise.

174. (B) 30-60.

As a general guideline, it is recommended that athletes consume approximately 30-60 grams of carbohydrates per hour before exercise.

175. (D) All of the options.

The correct answer is all of the options. Dehydration can occur if there is an imbalance of electrolytes in the body, which can lead to symptoms such as thirst, dry mouth, and fatigue. Muscle cramping is also a common symptom of an electrolyte imbalance, particularly if there is a deficiency of sodium, calcium, or magnesium. Finally, an electrolyte imbalance can also affect cognitive function and lead to confusion or disorientation.

176. (D) Creatine.

Creatine is not a stimulant commonly used in long-duration exercises that necessitate short bursts of energy. However, Caffeine, ephedrine, and cocaine are all stimulants that have been used by athletes to enhance performance during long-duration exercises that require short bursts of energy.

177. (D) Both A) and B)

The "two-for-two" rule suggests that the load should be increased if an individual can perform two additional repetitions for two consecutive workouts, and the load should be decreased if an individual cannot perform the desired number of repetitions for two consecutive workouts.

178. (A) ATP.

The principal source of energy for a muscular contraction is ATP (adenosine triphosphate). ATP is the energy currency of cells and is used to power many cellular processes, including muscle contraction.

179. (A) Cortisol.

Out of the options given, cortisol is the hormone that has the most significant influence on neural changes. Cortisol is a stress hormone that is released in response to stress, and it can have significant effects on the brain and neural function.

180. (B) Cortisol.

At rest, women typically have higher levels of cortisol compared to men. Cortisol is a steroid hormone that is produced by the adrenal gland in response to stress, and it plays a role in regulating many physiological processes, including metabolism, immune function, and the stress response.

181. (D) Testicular atrophy.

Testicular atrophy is a potential side effect of anabolic steroid use in men. Other potential side effects of anabolic steroid use in men may include breast enlargement (gynecomastia), deepened voice, and increased body hair growth. However, these side effects are not as common as testicular atrophy.

182. (B) 30 seconds.

The recommended rest period between sets during a high-intensity interval training (HIIT) workout is generally 30 seconds to 1 minute.

183. (C) 4.

The snatch is an Olympic lift consisting of four fundamental components executed as a single fluid lift.

184. (A) Increased compressive force on joints.

Increased compressive force on joints is a reason why athletes weighing over 220 pounds may be more susceptible to injury during plyometric exercises.

185. (B) Increased heart rate and blood pressure.

Increased heart rate and blood pressure best describe a person's physiological response to acute stress. When a person experiences acute stress, the body's sympathetic nervous system is activated, leading to a "fight or flight" response. This response is characterized by an increase in heart rate, blood pressure, and respiration rate.

186. (A) Eustress is a positive feeling of stress, while distress is a negative feeling of stress.

The difference between eustress and distress is that eustress is a positive feeling of stress, while distress is a negative feeling of stress. Eustress refers to a type of stress that is experienced as a positive feeling, such as the excitement and anticipation that someone may feel before a challenging task or event. Distress, on the other hand, refers to a type of stress that is experienced as a negative feeling, such as anxiety, fear, or frustration.

187. (D) None of the options.

Hips being too high at the start of the crouch position, stepping out laterally during the initial drive phase, and jumping the first stride or stepping over the knee of the stance leg are all common errors in sprinting technique. So the correct option is D.

188. (A) Selective attention.

The correct answer is selective attention. The athlete in this scenario is most likely using selective attention to concentrate solely on her performance and ignore the audience. Selective attention is the ability to focus on specific stimuli while ignoring others, and it is often used by athletes to block out distractions and maintain their focus on the task at hand.

189. (C) Prioritize isolation exercises over compound exercises.

The incorrect statement about the general basics of selecting exercise is: "Prioritize isolation exercises over compound exercises." The general recommendation is to prioritize compound exercises over isolation exercises. When selecting an exercise, it is recommended to start with the basics, such as multi-joint exercises before single-joint exercises, prioritize exercises that are appropriate for your fitness level and goals, and consider any injuries or limitations that may require modifications or specific rehabilitation exercises.

190. (A) Median.

The measure of central tendency that would best describe the typical time taken to complete the sprint is the median. The median represents the middle value in a data set when the values are arranged in order. It is less affected by outliers or extreme values, which can skew the mean. In this case, the median time would represent the typical time taken to complete the sprint for the group of football players.

191. (B). Median.

The most appropriate measure of central tendency for a group with five scores that are much higher than the rest is the median. The median represents the middle value in a data set when the values are arranged in order, and it is less influenced by extreme values than the mean.

192. (A) Cast kettlebell.

The type of kettlebell in the options given is Cast kettlebell. The other options, "Dumbbell kettlebell," "Curl kettlebell," and "Farmer's kettlebell," are not recognized types of kettlebells.

193. (D) Time, if any, to pause between the concentric and eccentric portions of the exercise.

Therefore, the fourth digit in the tempo digit represents the time, if any, to pause between the concentric and eccentric portions of the exercise.

194. (C) A wide stance with the feet pointed outward.

The sumo lift is characterized by a wide stance with the feet pointed outward. In this lift, the lifter's feet are placed wider than shoulder-width apart, with the toes pointing outward at an angle of approximately 45 degrees.

195. (B) Standing upright with the feet shoulder-width apartThe proper starting position for a conventional deadlift is to stand upright with the feet shoulder-width apart. To perform a conventional deadlift, the lifter should approach the barbell and position their feet hip-width apart with their toes pointing forward.

196. (C). Maintaining a neutral spine.

The technique that can be used to prevent rounding of the back during the deadlift exercise is Maintaining a neutral spine. Rounding of the back can lead to increased stress on the spinal discs, which can cause injury. The answer is C.

197. (A) Failing to reach parallel.

A common technique error during the high-bar Olympic squat is failing to reach parallel. Failing to reach parallel means that the lifter is not lowering its hips to the appropriate depth. This error can be caused by mobility restrictions or poor technique, such as leaning too far forward or shifting the weight onto the toes.

198. (B) Bulgarian split squat.

The Bulgarian split squat is a unilateral lower-body exercise that is similar to the barbell back squat. This exercise is commonly performed with dumbbells, or a barbell held on the back, similar to a barbell back squat.

199. (A) Lateral lunge. The lateral lunge is commonly used to target the adductor muscles. The lateral lunge also targets the glutes, hamstrings, and quadriceps, making it an effective exercise for overall lower-body strength and stability.

200. (B) Standing overhead press.

The standing overhead press is a compound exercise that targets multiple muscle groups, including the chest, shoulders, and triceps. Hence the correct answer is B.

201. (D) None of the options.

All of the factors listed, including differences in body type, muscular strength, and power output, can affect exercise techniques. Hence Option D is correct.

202. (C) Male pattern baldness.

Male pattern baldness is not a psychological factor that affects athlete performance. The other factors listed can all have an impact on an athlete's performance. For example, depression can affect an athlete's motivation, energy levels, and ability to focus, while increased aggressiveness and anger can either help or hinder performance depending on the situation.

203. (D) All of the options.

All of the options depict the effect of alcohol on athlete performance. Alcohol can impair motor skills, decrease coordination, and impair balance, which can have a negative impact on athletic performance. Additionally, alcohol can also impair cognitive function, decrease reaction time, and cause dehydration, all of which can further affect an athlete's performance. This is why it is generally recommended that athletes avoid consuming alcohol before or during athletic events.

204. (C) Body composition.

Basal metabolic rate (BMR) is primarily determined by an individual's body composition, specifically the amount of lean body mass (muscle mass). Individuals with a higher percentage of lean body mass tend to have a higher BMR, as muscle tissue is more metabolically active than fat tissue. Other factors, such as age, gender, and activity level, can also influence BMR, but body composition has the most significant impact.

205. (D) I, II, and III.

The correct answer is (I, II, and III). Iron is an important nutrient for athletes as it is involved in the production of hemoglobin, which carries oxygen to the muscles. Adequate iron intake can increase oxygen uptake and improve endurance during exercise. Iron can also have a positive effect on heart rate, as it is involved in the production of red blood cells, which carry oxygen to the muscles and help to regulate heart rate. In addition, iron has been shown to lower lactate concentrations during exercise, which can reduce muscle fatigue and improve exercise performance.

206. (A) Creatine

Creatine is known to increase hydration. Creatine is a naturally occurring compound found in small amounts in certain foods and produced by the body. It is stored primarily in the muscles and plays a crucial role in the production of energy during high-intensity exercises. When supplementing with creatine, it increases the amount of creatine phosphate stored in the muscles, which in turn helps to produce more adenosine triphosphate (ATP) during high-intensity workouts. This process leads to improved performance, strength, and power output.

207. (C) Rear deltoid fly.

The rear deltoid fly primarily targets the posterior deltoid, as it involves horizontal shoulder abduction, the primary function of the posterior deltoid.

208. (B) I and II.

The correct answer is (I and II) - both the antidiuretic hormone (ADH) and the renin-angiotensin-aldosterone system (RAAS) maintain electrolyte and water homeostasis during exercise. During exercise, the body's fluid balance can be disrupted by sweating and changes in blood flow, which can lead to dehydration and electrolyte imbalances. ADH helps to counteract these effects by increasing water reabsorption and reducing urine output, which helps to maintain electrolyte and water balance in the body. Similarly, the RAAS system helps regulate blood pressure and fluid balance in the body by controlling the levels of the hormone aldosterone, which promotes sodium and water retention by the kidneys.

209. (B) Rumination disorder.

The condition where a person regurgitates partially digested food and either re-chews, re-swallows, or discards it is called rumination disorder. Therefore, option (B) is the correct answer.

210. (D) Vitamin B.

Vitamin B is a water-soluble vitamin. Water-soluble vitamins are those that dissolve in water and are not stored in the body to any significant extent. In contrast, vitamins A, E, and K are fat-soluble vitamins, which means that they are absorbed and stored in fat cells in the body. Therefore, option (B) is the correct answer.

211. (B) It provides the quick bursts of energy required for speed.

The statement "It provides the quick bursts of energy required for speed" is false about fats. Other options are correct. Fat is the primary fuel source for light to moderate-intensity exercise. It is recommended that 10% of fat intake come from monounsaturated sources and that athletes should consume 20-35% of their total daily calories as fat. Therefore, option (B) is the correct answer.

212. (D) Jellies.

Jellies are a simple carbohydrate. Simple carbohydrates are composed of one or two sugar units and are quickly digested and absorbed by the body, leading to a rapid increase in blood sugar levels. Jellies are typically made from sugar and contain little to no fiber, protein, or fat, making them a source of quick energy but providing little nutritional value. In contrast, whole-grain bread, bagels, and brown rice are complex carbohydrates.

213. (D) Adequate Intake (AI).

Adequate Intake (AI) is a level assumed to ensure nutritional adequacy when there is insufficient evidence to develop a Recommended Dietary Allowance (RDA). On the other hand, The Recommended Dietary Allowance (RDA) is the average daily intake level that is sufficient to meet the nutrient requirements of nearly all healthy individuals in a particular life stage and gender group. Hence option D is correct.

214. (B) Pectoralis major and deltoid.

The muscles affected by the stretch in which one arm is pulled across the chest and held in position with the other arm are the pectoralis major and deltoid muscles. When the arm is pulled across the chest and held in position with the other arm, it stretches the pectoralis major muscle, which is the large muscle in the front of the chest, and the anterior fibers of the deltoid muscle, which is a muscle that covers the shoulder joint.

215. (B) Barbells and dumbbells.

For performing the bench press and forward step lunge exercises, the barbells, and dumbbells as the most appropriate equipment. Barbells and dumbbells provide versatile and adjustable resistance that can be easily increased or decreased to accommodate various fitness levels and goals.

216. (D) Weightlifting.

Using a spotter is recommended for weightlifting exercises. Weightlifting exercises typically involve lifting heavy weights, which can put a lot of stress on the body and increase the risk of injury, especially if proper form is not maintained or if the lifter becomes fatigued. A spotter can help the lifter safely lift and lower the weight, provide feedback on form, and assist in case the lifter is unable to complete the lift.

217. (C) Directly above the bar.

When an athlete pulls weight from the floor in a deadlift, the shoulders should be in front of the bar. In a deadlift, the bar should be pulled in a straight line from the floor to the standing position. To achieve this, the shoulders should be directly above or slightly in front of the bar at the start of the lift.

218. (A) Pronated grip.

To minimize the assistance of the biceps brachii muscle, a weightlifter should use a pronated grip for the lat pull-down exercise. A pronated grip, also known as an overhand grip, involves holding the bar with palms facing away from the body and fingers wrapped around the bar.

219. (C) On the lifter's wrists.

When spotting someone for a dumbbell shoulder press or bench press, the spotter's hands should be on the lifter's wrists. This allows the spotter to assist the lifter in lifting the weight, while also providing stability and control to prevent the weight from dropping on the lifter's face or chest.

220. (A) Creatine.

Creatine is a performance-enhancing supplement that is not currently classified as a controlled substance and can be purchased as a legal dietary supplement. Cocaine and erythropoietin are both illegal substances that are not approved for use as performance-enhancing drugs. Ephedrine was previously used in dietary supplements for weight loss and energy enhancement, but it is now regulated by the FDA and is only available by prescription or as a limited-use ingredient in certain dietary supplements. Hence, the correct answer is A.